HAIR

UNTANGLING A
SOCIAL HISTORY

Library of Congress Cataloging-in-Publication Data

Jolly, Penny Howell.
Hair : untangling a social history / Penny Howell Jolly ; with essays
by Gerald M. Erchak ... [et al.].
      p.   cm.
Catalog of an exhibition at the Frances Young Tang Teaching Museum and
Art Gallery at Skidmore College, Jan. 31–June 6, 2004.
Includes bibliographical references.
ISBN 0-9725188-3-5 (alk. paper)
1. Hair—Social aspects—Exhibitions. 2. Hair in art—Exhibitions.
3. Hairstyles—History—Exhibitions. 4. Frances Young Tang Teaching
Museum and Art Gallery—Exhibitions. I. Erchak, Gerald Michael. II.
Frances Young Tang Teaching Museum and Art Gallery. III. Skidmore
College. Art Gallery. IV. Title.
GT2290.J65 2004
391.6—dc22

2003026335

HAIR

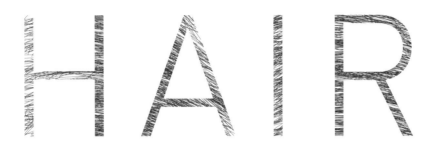

UNTANGLING A
SOCIAL HISTORY

Penny Howell Jolly

WITH ESSAYS BY

**Gerald M. Erchak, Amelia Rauser,
Jeffrey O. Segrave, and Susan Walzer**

THE FRANCES YOUNG TANG
TEACHING MUSEUM AND ART GALLERY
AT SKIDMORE COLLEGE

To Jay Rogoff, for all his help and support

7   **INTRODUCTION TO A SOCIAL HISTORY OF HAIR**
ROOTS, KNOTS, AND TANGLES
Penny Howell Jolly

13   ***HOMO HIRSUTUS***
THE EVOLUTION OF HUMAN HAIR GROWTH PATTERN
Gerald M. Erchak

21   **THE FASHIONABLE MAN**
Penny Howell Jolly

29   **SEX AND SENSIBILITY**
HAIR IN THE MACARONI CARICATURES OF THE 1770S
Amelia Rauser

39   **THE TROUBLE WITH LARRY**
SOCIAL MEANINGS OF MALE BALDNESS
Susan Walzer

47   **THE IDEAL WOMAN**
Penny Howell Jolly

59   **HAIR POWER**
Penny Howell Jolly

75   **(H)AIR JORDAN**
EXCAVATING HIS ROYAL BALDNESS
Jeffrey O. Segrave

85   PLATES

109   CONTRIBUTORS

110   SELECTED BIBLIOGRAPHY

112   EXHIBITION CHECKLIST

118   ACKNOWLEDGMENTS

120   CREDITS

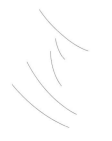

INTRODUCTION TO A SOCIAL HISTORY OF HAIR ROOTS, KNOTS, AND TANGLES

Penny Howell Jolly

WE WASH IT AND DRY IT, bleach it and dye it. It grows—where we want it and where we don't—and we curl and straighten it, shave and transplant it, grow it long or tweeze it, cover it with wigs and tame it with nets. We buy conditioners, wax treatments, wigs and switches, frosting kits, blow dryers, razors, curling irons, powders, and sprays. One person waxes his moustache, while another plucks and bleaches hers. Growth of body hair tells us we are mature, and its loss signals our decline.

Hair grows on select parts of our bodies, and we—like our ancestors before us—manipulate it to tell our world who we are. Before we say a word to a new acquaintance, our visible hair identifies us by announcing our gender, class, religion, or politics. Hair styles and body hair grooming form a semiotic system, creating a series of signs legible to those in our social groups. The meanings of these visual codes, of course, change over time and according to social context, and are more dependent upon *difference*—long vs. short, shaved vs. hirsute—than any system of stable meaning. Shifts in hair style typically reflect major political and social movements, as when hippies in the 1960s grew long hair and beards to separate their counterculture from the finely coiffed establishment, feminists in the 1970s stopped shaving legs and axillary (underarm) hair, and black men and women wore Afros to signal their return to their racial roots.

By nature, almost all humans have visible hair: on the tops of heads, as eyebrows and eyelashes, as axillary hair, and pubic hair. In addition, most areas of human skin produce hair, typically finer in women and more noticeable in men. Even in people of least hairy appearance, only a few areas of dermis are truly hairless (called glabrous skin):

fingertips, palms, soles of feet and toes, lips, nipples, and highly sensitive parts of the male and female genitalia. Some people are born totally or partially hairless, a condition called alopecia, while others have excessive hair all over their bodies: hypertrichosis. The cross-sectional shape of the hair shaft determines its texture: perfectly round hairs are straight and more coarse, oval ones are silky and wavy, while flatter shafts are kinky. Hair color is determined by the varied proportions of melanins of different color, called melanocytes, at the base of the hair follicle. Red hair, a recessive trait and the least common hair color (only 2–5 percent of humans worldwide), results from the presence of an iron compound; gray and white hair results from decreased melanin production and its replacement by air bubbles in the shaft. Typically, people start growing gray hairs in their twenties, and about half the population is gray by age fifty.

But no person's hair is truly "natural." In societies worldwide, differing social circumstances determine the appearance of head and body hair. For instance, religious institutions frequently control hair: Christian monks shave their head hair into tonsures and Muslim women cover theirs, while Hasidic men grow payis and their wives wear wigs in public. Hair styling also reinforces class and political differences. In France, powdered wigs initially distinguished seventeenth- and eighteenth-century aristocrats— giving rise to the term "bigwig"—but were then sported by the rising bourgeoisie, only to be finally overturned by the revolutionaries' assertion of republican "naturalism" following the Revolution. For Fidel Castro, the beard identified his followers, setting them apart from the defeated, clean-shaven Cuban army: "Your beard does not belong to you. It belongs to the Revolution."[1] Today neo-Nazi skinheads, by their almost bald pates, signal a return to fascist politics, and Hitler's Aryan blonde ideal is revived—an ideal which never existed within the actual German population of the 1930s.[2]

With rare exception, head and body hair styles work to exaggerate differences between the sexes rather than downplay them. While these physical differences between males and females are not in fixed opposition, social conventions work to make them distinct: in one era, men's hair may be longer and more elaborately dressed than women's—the lovelocks of seventeenth-century England or elaborate wig styles of early eighteenth-century France—while in another, the women's outshines the men's—as in Renaissance Italy, when women entwined and braided jewels in their hair, or in the early 1960s with the bouffant. When women's legs were suddenly visible due to 1920s fashions, they needed to differ from men's, and shaving became fashionable. Hair further distinguishes stages in the life cycle of both males and females, as moustaches and beards separate pre-adolescent boys from mature males, a biological difference; or, in a socially constructed difference, long, flowing hair marks the fertile virgin, ripe and ready for marriage, and distinguishes her from the properly married matron whose hair is bound up. When women began bobbing their hair in the 1920s, some men feared the end of all civilization, apparently associating flowing locks with actual fertility.

Hair color similarly carries meaning—consider the stereotypes of the "dumb" blonde and the sultry but unpredictable redhead—as does hair's overall form. Heinrich Hoffmann's moralizing children's book from 1845, *Struwwelpeter* (*Slovenly Peter*), offers cautionary tales that link proper grooming to proper behavior; Peter's wild hair and unclipped fingernails clearly reveal his naughtiness. Long, sinuous hair on a female signals her highly sexual nature, and metaphors abound of men being captured in its tangles, warning of the power of hair (and women) over men. Baldness in men has traditionally implied impotency. Hirsute Samson's loss at the hand of Delilah only reinforces that myth, as does the practice of cutting or shaving the hair of defeated foes—prisoners, enemy collaborators, concentration camp victims—as a sign of humiliation and subjection. Locks of hair, on the other hand, remain intimate reminders of absent loved ones.

Hair styling—for both women and men—does not come inexpensively, and supports a multibillion-dollar industry, including both hair salons and modern do-it-yourself home hair care products that have flooded the market to make change increasingly easy. Throughout history, formulas, equipment, and personnel for manipulating hair have flourished. Our exhibition, which focuses on the Renaissance to the present, demonstrates the ubiquitous nature of products and tools related to hair care. Particularly famous ad campaigns from the twentieth century are represented: the Gillette Company's invention of the safety razor, the Breck Girl campaign for shampoo, and Burma Shave's famous roadside jingles.

The essays in this volume treat a number of these issues in closer detail, and from a variety of disciplines. Gerald M. Erchak, in his "*Homo Hirsutus*: The Evolution of Human Hair Growth Pattern," approaches questions concerning the role of human hairiness in males and females from biological and anthropological perspectives. My own essay, "The Fashionable Man," considers ways that male humans manipulate their head and facial hair—the wig and the beard play important roles—to express identities and ideologies. Amelia Rauser's essay, "Sex and Sensibility: Hair in the Macaroni Caricatures of the 1770s," focuses on satirical prints of the eighteenth century, exploring how hair functioned as a signifier in the visual arts, specifically for figures of the foppish macaroni. Using a sociological perspective, Susan Walzer explores the loss of head hair (and self-esteem) in men in "The Trouble with Larry: Social Meanings of Male

Baldness." Is it better to be authentically bald, or to cover up with a comb-over, transplant, or toupee?

In the subsequent essay, I trace "The Ideal Woman" from the Renaissance to modern times, interrogating why fashions change and why some ideals—such as the blonde—remain relatively consistent. My "Hair Power" essay then turns more specifically to sexually potent hair, to meanings attributed to body hair, to the role of hair in memory and mourning, and finally to the importance of hair in African-American experience. Michael Jordan's shaved African-American head is the multi-layered subject of the final essay in this volume, Jeffrey O. Segrave's "(H)Air Jordan: Excavating His Royal Baldness." Segrave's analysis ranges broadly from consideration of racial and sociopolitical issues in America today to sports, consumerism, and marketing.

1. Quoted by David Kunzle in *Che Guevara* (Los Angeles: UCLA Fowler Museum, 1997), 49. I thank Jennifer Jolly for this reference.

2. On Nazi "race science" and blondeness, see Pat Shipman, *The Evolution of Racism* (New York: Simon and Schuster, 1994), especially chapter 8; and Joanna Pitman, *On Blondes* (London: Bloomsbury, 2003), especially 155–165 and 183–201.

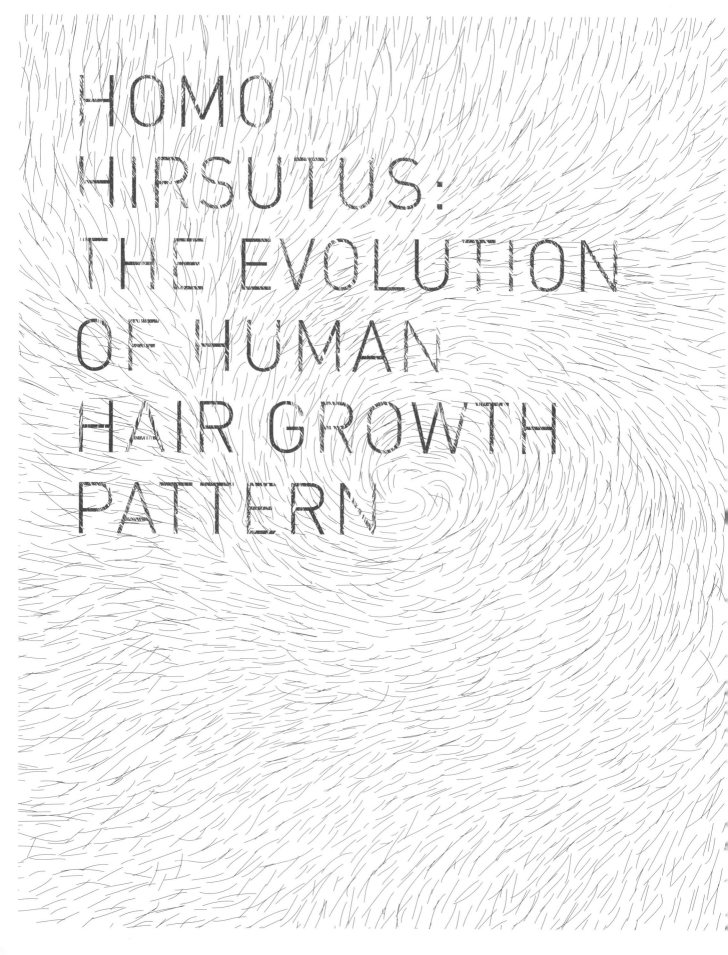

Gerald M. Erchak

And when her days to be delivered were fulfilled,
behold, there were twins in her womb.
And the first came out red, all over like an hairy garment;
And they called his name Esau.
(Gen. 25:24–25)

And Jakob said to Rebekah his mother,
Behold, Esau my brother is a hairy man,
and I am a smooth man.
(Gen. 27:11)

JACOB THEN WENT ON TO BE THE PROGENITOR of the twelve tribes of Israel, while Esau ruled over the Edomites who, as far as I can tell, have not survived the march of history. In the Bible, Esau is a hunter and outdoorsman, a man of the open plains, while Jacob is a villager, a settled farmer: barbarian vs. civilized, as it were. Jacob is favored by his mother, while Esau is favored by his father, Isaac. Jacob consistently wins over Esau, stealing his birthright, getting his father's blessing meant for Esau, and so on. This would seem to be a clear biblical warning about the negative effects of hairiness.

Indeed humans were once upon a time hairy beasts, or at least our ancestors were. Now, with some exceptions—like Alec Baldwin, Robin Williams, and perhaps, Frida Kahlo—we are smooth. Why did we lose our body hair? And why have we retained the body hair that we have?

Zoologists will quite rightly say that we haven't lost our hair. We still have as many hairs as we did millions of years ago; it's just that each hair has shrunk to a fine light downiness, as if, in the words of Jonathan Kingdon, "baby down was stopped from growing into an adult pelt. Our hair became puny and almost invisible, giving the illusion of hairlessness."[1] While this is certainly true, I will focus on *visible* body hair.

For the most part, I will examine the current state of our hair in terms of evolution, especially that process Darwin named sexual selection, although other aspects of hair pattern and evolution—for example, natural selection—will also be considered. In this process, sexual selection, males and females develop certain traits not so much because they help them survive in their environments on a day-to-day basis, but rather because they help them attract mates and reproduce. The classic example is the peacock's tail, useless for procuring food or shelter, useless for defense—in fact at some point, were the tail larger, it would be ultimately fatal. However, it makes the male supremely attractive to the peahen, probably as an indicator or signal of good health, good genes, good mating material.

Why did we lose much of our body hair in the course of evolution, but keep it on the top of the head? I should note here that I will not really consider baldness, nor nostril hairs, nor eyebrows nor lashes, nor that peculiar old-age male phenomenon of hair growing out of, and on, the ears. (I should mention, however, that very recently B. Y. Tyagi of Bhopal, India, has claimed the title of longest ear hair in the world, at four inches! Not very impressive, really.) In any case, these will remain unanalyzed. I would venture that the earhairs business, at least, resists adaptational explanation, unless anyone here can come up with a reason why burgeoning ear hair in sixty-year-old men enhances survival! No, these things occur post-reproduction, and are therefore outside of my envelope of discourse.

Back to the head. A lack of body hair is most conspicuous in the tropics, suggesting a link between human nakedness and coolness. Hairiness makes sweating less effective. As Kingdon notes, a person can sweat as much as 28 litres in twenty-four hours in a hot climate. "It is clearly preferable that such salts and wastes should wash off rather than build up in a mat of hair."[2] But hair on the head is really important in the tropics. Africans, despite being the most hairless of peoples, have the densest and most matted hair of all humans—on their heads. Their spiral hair, a later development from the original straight hair, creates a thick protective shield over the brain, essential for diurnal tropical hunters. The brain must be kept at a constant temperature.

Our lack of noticeable body hair is an example of neoteny, an anthropological term for the extension of childlike characteristics into adulthood. Our neotenous hairlessness is a childlike characteristic unknown among other primates. Let's spend a minute looking at our hairlessness before looking at our hairiness. The late great anthropologist Ashley Montagu, in a wonderful book entitled *The Natural Superiority of Women*, notes that humans as they grow remain more like an infant than does the ape; for example, the skull of an infant gorilla more closely resembles the skull of an adult human than it does an adult gorilla.[3] In other words, the adult human being is an infantilized or pedomorphic type, a type that has evolved by preserving some youthful ancestral characteristics, while the gorilla is an aged or gerontomorphic type, a type that has evolved by accentuated development of already adult characteristics. Provocatively, yet a bit obviously, he notes that the human female skull more closely resembles that of an infant than does the male skull. Thus, the human female maintains the evolutionary promise of the infant skull more than does the male and is thus in the evolutionary vanguard while the male falls somewhat behind. He goes on to argue that humans are even fetus-like, rather than infant-like, and that of all peoples the most fetus-like—and, he's suggesting, the "best-evolved"—are the Chinese. In other words, the infant type is the type toward which human development is directed, and human evolution has actually come about as a result of the slowing up of our development, in the womb as well as after birth. "The developmental promise of the human infant is more fully realized by the female than by the male"[4]—not only in her hairlessness, including the face, but in her less protuberant brow ridges, smoother bones, softer skin, different torso-to-leg ratio, and so forth. I don't want to belabor this point, but Montagu is saying that in this special sense women are "more evolved," a phrase I know will make biologists weep. Montagu quotes the eighteenth-century German poet Schiller: "*Aus der bezaubernden Anmut der Zuge Leuchtet der Menschheit Vollendung und Wiege*" (From the bewitching gracefulness of the features shines forth the fulfillment of humanity).[5] Within American culture, women further emphasize and maintain their relative hairlessness by shaving "412 inches of their bodies 11 times a month."[6]

As the character Elaine Bennis once said on *Seinfeld*, "Men's bodies are functional, simian; women's are works of art." So men are more ape-like. Perhaps Montagu's notions help us understand why pop star Jon Bon Jovi and tennis star Andre Agassi have famously shaved their chests in recent years, erasing "the stigma of Esau." In fact, according to the makers of Nair, in 2001, "30 percent of men aged 18 to 34 regularly shaved their chests."[7] Whether the new appeal of hairy-chested stalwart "manly men" in the wake of the 9/11 disaster and the elevation of police and firefighters in the public sexual aesthetic reverse this pro-androgyny or "Jacobean" trend remains to be seen.[8]

What about beards? Why don't women have them? Sexual selection operates on males especially in the area of male-male competition. Men would not want to look neotenous—like a child or a woman. The beard takes care of that. In addition, it de-individuates the man, masking his features and accentuating his fierceness. It makes the head appear larger. As Darwin wrote, "Our male ape-like progenitors acquired their beards as an ornament to charm or excite the opposite sex." Anthropologist Helen Fisher suggests that men retained their chest hair for the same reason, and goes on to argue that females lost their facial and chest hair to expose the sensitive areas around the mouth and breast, facilitating sexual stimulation. "Without a thick mat of hair she could display puckered sensual lips and bulging breasts to excite a potential mate."[9] Jonathan Kingdon argues that "beards are a visual device to enlarge the face," to impress women and to impress rival men.[10] Selection in favor of beards reflects prehistoric preferences: sophisticated modern cultures promote shaving or neat trimming to erase this reminder of prehistoric unruliness. The average American man, according to the Gillette Company, shaves "an area of 48 square inches 24 times a month."[11] However, some other cultures do want to maintain a firm facial distinction between men and women, and these cultures promote moustaches. Of course, there is a great deal of variation, with Native American and Asian men having very little facial hair, in contrast to the heavy beards of many European and Japanese Ainu males.

Let us now move down below the neck. Let me say straightaway that there is no relationship between amount of body hair and adaptation to cold, as even the most cursory comparison of people around the globe will show. Kingdon notes that "it is uncertain when and why people became 'naked' but selectively 'tufted' on top of the head, over the brows, in the groin, and under the arms."[12] One theory argues that body hair is related to sex, that is, to sex differences and to sexuality. It is related to the senses of sight, smell, and touch. Remember we are speaking of a prehistoric world in which everyone is nude all the time. The appearance of body hair on the developing child is a visible recognizable sign to the community that the individual is ready for sex and reproduction. For boys, pubic hair appears around the time of genital development and facial and axillary hair a year or two later. For girls, pubic hair usually appears shortly after breast growth begins. Note that in the past—in fact, even in the not-so-distant past—these signs appeared several years later than they do today.

The greater hairiness of the male, or the greater hairlessness of the human female, also evolved to intensify and clarify—and announce to the community and anyone around, along with other signs of sexual dimorphism—that the individual is indeed a man or a woman. Such clarity was important in the completely non-androgynous times of the Paleolithic.

In addition to being a sign of sexual maturity and sex difference, body hair is patterned as it is in order to concentrate and diffuse body odors, specifically pheromones, into the air more readily. Apocrine glands are the major source of human odor, and the location of these glands coincides with the main areas where hair is retained: on the chest, under the arms, around the navel, around the genitals, and around the anus.[13] And scent may play an important role in sexual stimulation. With face-to-face supine intercourse, the partners are closer and scent can become a relevant sexual stimulus. Apocrine glands secrete the odorous component of sweat when humans are either frightened or sexually stimulated. They are heavily concentrated under the arms and in the so-called erogenous zones. Anthropologist Suzanne Frayser speculates that subtle scents may reinforce a tendency to pay particular attention to stimulating these areas. Since males are more likely than females to produce a discernible odor from these glands, they may be giving females information about the degree of their partner's sexual excitement, thus providing another criterion for sexual selection. A chemical called androstenol is found in male sweat, and its dry musty smell is appealing to women. When it oxidizes, it forms androstenone, the smell of which women tend to react negatively to, unless they are ovulating. A similar synthetic substance, alpha androstenol, when sniffed by sows causes them to go into lordosis, that is, to adopt the mating position of presenting the posterior. While scientists have not demonstrated such an effect on human females, there are other suggestive experimental findings about the role of human pheromones, called by some "copulins" or "copulines," wafted as they are into the air by body hair. For example, when a "donor" woman wears cotton pads under her arms for a twenty-four-hour period and other women are then exposed to her armpit odor, the menstrual periods of the recipient women shift to become closer to the periods of the donor. In another study, women who seldom dated men had longer cycles; women who often dated men had shorter and more regular cycles. Women who had slept with men once a week were more likely to have regular menstrual cycles and fewer fertility problems. The cause was not sexual activity *per se*, since masturbation made no difference. The man's underarm odor is what made the difference. It has been found that armpit secretions from men mixed with alcohol and dabbed on the upper lip of women will also regularize their periods almost as effectively.[14] Despite our diligent efforts to eliminate and conceal these odors, they may still be part of the silent language of sex.

Most recently, Jonathan Kingdon argues that hairlessness helped us "combat skin disease and parasites."[15] When early humans began to spend greater amounts of time in their encampments, human waste would build up, along with parasites and disease-carrying animals; "bacterial, fungal, and viral infections sheltered by a soiled hairy cover and provided with a purchase via glands attached to the abundant roots" would disadvantage hairier people over the less hairy. Sebaceous glands are most directly related to hair, and are especially dense around the anus, genitals, mouth, and eyes where "they probably help inhibit infection."[16]

Those are some possible suggestions why we are hairy, but the evolution of the human species involved our becoming progressively and neotenously more hairless. And this is where the sense of touch comes in, where our exquisitely sensitive fingertips and lips meet the now-hairless skin of our mates. "With the loss of thick body hair, later in human evolution, the general nakedness of human bodies exposed more areas of the skin, which could be stimulated by touch," according to Suzanne Frayser, who goes on to say "The skin may well be our largest sex organ."[17] Primates derive great pleasure from grooming each other, and our ability to directly stimulate the skin extends this pleasure. So the loss of visible body hair had a sexual advantage, exposing the soft delicate areas of the neck, abdomen, and legs. A touch to these areas could now arouse one's partner to intercourse. In addition, these areas could now be seen, especially during frontal copulation. As Helen Fisher describes it, "When a female blushed, her partner knew she was responding to his touch or speech. When a female's nipples hardened, her partner was informed that she was getting sexually excited. And the sexual flush that occurs during orgasm was obvious to both."[18] The loss of visible body hair enabled partners to signal their desire, to express their excitement, to arouse each other with touch and sight—a tremendous service at a time when sex had become important to survival.

1. Jonathan Kingdon, *Self-Made Man: Human Evolution from Eden to Extinction?* (New York: John Wiley & Sons, 1993), 244.

2. Kingdon, *Self-Made Man*, 244.

3 Ashley Montagu, *The Natural Superiority of Women* (New York: Collier Books, 1974), 70.

4. Montagu, 71.

5. Montagu, 73.

6. "The Rise of Mammals: Taking it on the Chin," *National Geographic Magazine*, April 2003, 140.

7. Zarah Crawford, "Bear Market," *Men's Fashions of the Times*, 22 September 2002, 90.

8. Crawford, "Bear Market," 90, 92.

9. Helen Fisher, *Anatomy of Love* (New York: Fawcett Columbine, 1999), 99.

10. Kingdon, *Self-Made Man*, 233.

11. "The Rise of Mammals," 140.

12. Kingdon, *Lowly Origin: Where, When, and Why Our Ancestors First Stood Up* (Princeton, N.J.: Princeton University Press, 2003), 325.

13. Suzanne G. Frayser, *Varieties of Sexual Experience: An Anthropological Perspective on Human Sexuality* (New Haven: HRAF Press, 1985) 61; Kingdon, Lowly Origin, 326.

14. Meredith F. Small, *What's Love Got to Do with It? The Evolution of Human Mating* (New York: Doubleday, 1995), 73–76.

15. Kingdon, *Lowly Origin*, 325.

16. Kingdon, *Lowly Origin*, 326.

17. Frayser, *Varieties of Sexual Experience*, 61.

18. Fisher, *Anatomy of Love*, 98.

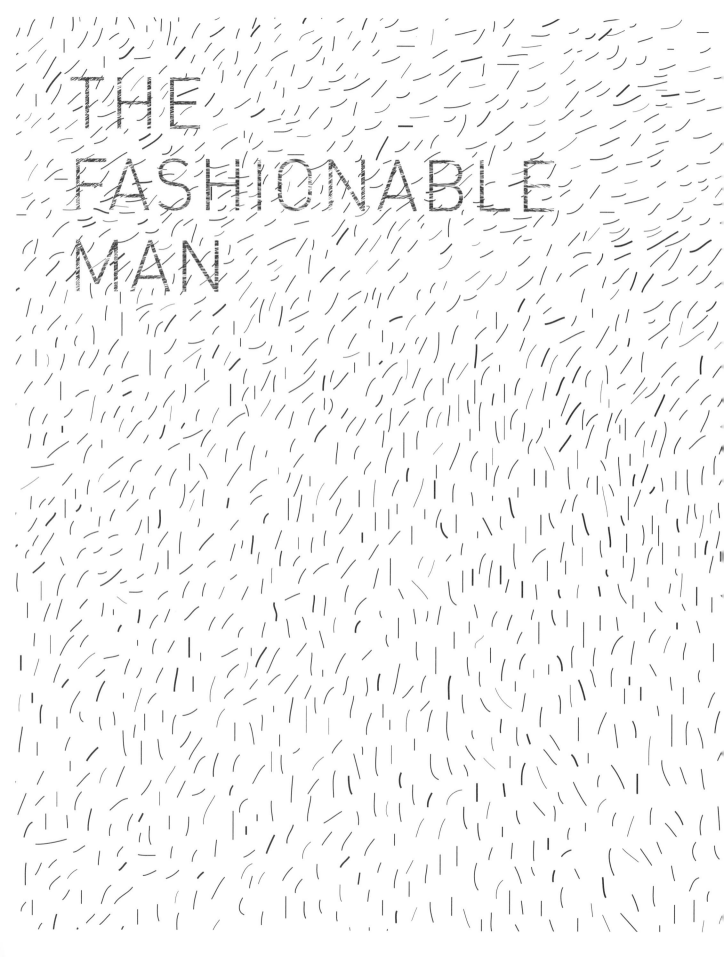

Penny Howell Jolly

IT IS ERRONEOUS TO BELIEVE only women think about their hair. Much of people's concept of masculinity revolves around hair, whether head, facial, or body; thus throughout history, men have devoted significant time and energy to it. Today, one out of every twelve men colors his hair, whether to cover gray or "add excitement" to a tedious life (and 57 percent of women surveyed say this is fine with them). Among male teens and twenty-somethings, Bleach Blond, Sandstorm, Black Jack, and Red Rum are the currently popular dyes. And the men's hair coloring industry consumed $200 million in 2001.

Changes in personal grooming—women's and men's—are subject to fashion, and fashion responds to many factors. For example, the French aristocrat (probably the Count d'Angoulême) in the circa 1560 *Portrait* attributed to Corneille de Lyon (plate 4) wears his hair short-cropped, but along with a moustache and short, square-cut beard. The newly desirable short hair on males, not fashionable in the preceding century, arose from an accident to Francis I, King of France, in the 1520s: when the injury required his hair to be shaved, he demanded his entire court be shorn. This new French style spread quickly, as demonstrated by Henry VIII's English court, as did another newly fashionable display of hair—the beard. In previous centuries, beards differentiated foreigners, especially Easterners, from Europeans. But the beard's introduction following Francis I's accident may have served as a compensation for the lack of head hair, and its meaning was quickly established, making it indispensable. The Renaissance beard, popular beginning about 1540 and in vogue for at least a century, carried specific connotations regarding masculinity.[1]

As confirmed by medical treatises and essayists, as well as English poets and dramatists who punned on "hair" and "heir," hair in general and the beard specifically, once head hair was shorter, signified the wearer's virility. It was believed that the beard's hair was linked specifically to the production of semen. As Marcus Ulmus's treatise on beards declares, "Nature gave to mankind a Beard, that it might remaine as an Index in the Face, of the Masculine generative faculty."[2] According to the ancient theory of the humors, men were superior due to their naturally hot and dry natures, while women were cold and wet. Being without beard resulted from lack of heat: "Because they [women] want heate, as it appeareth also in some effeminate men, who are beardles for the same cause, because they are of the complexion of women."[3] On the other hand, and quite inconsistently, women's excessive head hair was understood to result from their cold, moist temperaments, as did their small and inferior brains. Thus, like the rational brains produced by men's hot natures, beards additionally indicated wisdom. Social circumstances also intervened, adding further prestige to beards: Elizabeth I of England set a tax on beards, effectively limiting them to upper-class males.[4] In modern times, beards still connote authority and influence: the CIA plotted to poison Fidel Castro's cigars in hopes of depilating and simultaneously deposing him.[5]

Men's hair fashions changed dramatically when eight-year-old Louis XIII ascended the French throne in 1610. His beardless face and long curly hair, parted in the middle, began the new fashion that quickly spread beyond France's borders. Following premature hair loss by the 1620s, Louis donned artificial hair and wigs in order to maintain the new fashion; his own scraggly beard led him in 1628 to limit his court's facial hair to moustaches and tiny chin tufts. Louis XIV continued the rage for long, elaborate hair, and when his "natural glory" began to thin at about age thirty-five, he similarly turned to hairpieces and wigs, employing as many as forty wigmakers; in 1665 the guild of wigmakers was established.

The English court followed French fashion, but already at James I's court there were complaints: "Men wearing long haire like vnto women, and women cutting off their haire like vnto boyes…. Oh monstrous, oh monstrous."[6] However, English courtiers enthusiastically adopted the French *cadenette*, or lovelock, an extra long curl of hair—or even five or six—usually falling over the left shoulder, the side "closer" to the heart; sometimes ribbons or jewels, love tokens offered by a lady, were attached. Cornelius Johnson's portrait from 1633 (plate 3), probably of Sir Francis Godolphin, depicts one of Charles I's courtiers in fashionable doublet with elaborate lace collar. Typical of English gentlemen up until the 1660s—when wigs became fashionable—his long hair is his own; the low collar allows his stylish lovelock to hang over his shoulder.

Associated with fashionable Royalists, lovelocks and long hair became sites for political as well as religious and moral controversy. The lovelock was trammeled by moralizing Christian writers for its effeminacy and degeneracy. William Prynne, in his 1628 *The Unlovelinesse, of Love-lockes. Or A summarie Discourse, prooving: The wearing, and nourishing of a Locke, or Love-locke, to be altogether unseemely, and unlawfull unto Christians*, not only condemned men for "the Womanish, Sinfull, and Unmanly, Crisping, Curling, Frouncing, Powdring, and nourishing of their Lockes, and Hairie excrements," but also took the opportunity to criticize women's "whorish Cutting and Crisping of their Haire... the very badge and character of their subjection both to God and Man."[7] The religious split became political as "Round-Heads"—a term first applied during the winter of 1641–1642 to Puritans and other supporters of Parliament who typically wore short, conservative haircuts—were at odds with the long-haired "Cavaliers," the sometimes raffish supporters of the King.[8] A pastor named Thomas Hall printed his *Loathsomnesse of Long Haire* in 1653, wherein he stated that "long haire is one of the sinfull customes and fashion of the wicked men of the world."[9] Similar pronouncements appear in the New England Colonies: in 1655 Harvard University outlawed long hair, and Massachusetts pastor Nicholas Noyes (1647–1717) wrote "An Essay Against Periwigs," wherein he condemned wigs while pondering significant questions regarding boundaries between young and old, women and men, humans and animals.[10] Nonetheless, Samuel Pepys succumbed to wearing a long-haired periwig in 1663, although when his wife attached extra locks to her hair, he forbade her the practice. But Pepys was no Puritan. While some women did sport periwigs, generally speaking wigs were articles of male dress and, like the Renaissance beard, signified masculinity and authority, connotations still alive today in England's judicial and political systems.[11]

Elaborately powdered wigs worn over fully clean-shaven faces continued in popularity into the eighteenth century (plate 7), although the problems caused by insects (the powder used was often flour) and fear of spreading the plague did discourage some. Wigs also became objects of political and social satire. William Hogarth's 1761 engraving, *The Five Orders of Periwigs* (plate 5), parodies Vitruvius's famous treatise on architectural orders, and simultaneously mocks the aristocracy by highlighting the pretentiousness surrounding wigs' authority and importance. His 1732–1733 *A Midnight Modern Conversation* (plate 21) shows a bawdy group of so-called gentlemen at a drinking house, a number of whom have lost their wigs and thus have symbolically shed civilization itself. Even here in the colonies, proper wigs conveyed orderliness and control, as documented in portraits of American merchant class families (plate 6). Men carefully balanced pious Puritan complaints against wigs with their desires to demonstrate prosperity and upward mobility. Thus male wigs needed to be appropriately modest in style, befitting conservative American society, and most colonial women dressed their natural hair, avoiding wigs altogether (plate 24).[12] Some men eschewed wigs entirely. George Washington (plate 34) refused to wear them, a practice too aristocratic for him, and was dismayed that Martha, a wealthy woman when he married her, was ordering wigs from abroad.

Economics and politics put an end to fanciful periwigs. In England in 1795, a famine year, Pitt's Tory government imposed a tax on flour for hair, and their opposition Whigs promptly cut off their pigtails and ceased powdering; powdered heads quickly went out of fashion. In France in the 1790s, supporters of the Revolution distinguished themselves from the establishment by eschewing wigs and returning to short, more natural hairstyles based on ancient Roman styles, as seen in Roman republican portrait busts and some later imperial images. Apparently inspired by an actor playing the role of Titus, Napoleon and others popularized this new "à la Titus" cut, which allowed for short, loose, lightly curled hair combed forward over the temples and forehead, and down the neck; finally dark colors, especially black hair, were in style. Established first in France, the now fashionable Titus cut spread across Europe to England and on to the newly formed United States. We see this, for example, in Thomas Sully's *Portrait of Tom Wharton* (plate 8) from the first decade of the nineteenth century. Even here there are political overtones to the new style, as, for example, followers of Thomas Jefferson cut their hair to contrast with the long-haired Federalists.[13]

While fashionable men's hair remained relatively short for the duration of the nineteenth century, countless portraits document the return of facial hair. Moustaches, beards, and even elaborate sideburns appear, the latter a popular style named after Ambrose Burnside, a Union general during the Civil War, who originated the fashion in the United States (plate 9).[14] This hirsute style coincides with the sale of numerous hair preparations promising luxuriant growth of hair and related products such as dyes and curling irons for whiskers and moustaches (plate 10).

But an enormous change occurred within the following two decades. Already by the sixteenth century, men had typically been shaven either at home by servants, or in public barbershops by barbers using a straight-edged razor (plate 12). Not until the early nineteenth century was there a serious movement afoot to encourage self-shaving by creating a so-called safety razor: an instrument where the skin was shielded from all but the edge of the blade. Finally, in 1895, in this country, King C. Gillette invented a safety razor with a pre-sharpened, disposable, one-use-only blade: man's morning *toilette* was now revolutionized. The patent was granted in 1903 and production began; by 1905, 90,000 razors and 2.5 million blades were produced and sold here and in Britain. It is estimated that today North American males spend an average of 3,000 hours shaving during their lifetimes—about four months of their lives.[15]

The twentieth century, then, is the period of increasing "do-it-yourself" options regarding hair. Gillette's enormously popular safety razor and those of competitors were instantly widely used. One company marketed a sharpenable blade where a strop was pulled through the razor alongside the blade's edge; such variants are on display in this exhibition. World War I helped to familiarize young men with the new tool, as safety razors were issued to soldiers, allowing them to maintain a clean-shaven face on the battlefield (plate 11). This was not an aesthetic decision; helmets and gas masks, for example, fit much better over smooth, hairless faces and chins. Throughout the century blades improved: carbon steel was replaced by stainless steel blades, and double- and triple-track razors were invented. The barbershop, once a place for political discussion and man-to-man social interaction, became a place for only infrequent visits.

Jacob Schick in 1923 patented the first electric razor, which—after a number of modifications—moved into significant use during the 1930s. In our exhibit is a highly successful competitor from 1925, the "New Improved Vibro-Shave" (plate 13). It looks like a normal double-edge safety razor, but plugs in, using electricity to vibrate the blade in its head. The so-called "dry razor," requiring no water source or lather, developed throughout the rest of the century. On the brink of World War II, companies like Remington and Sunbeam joined in to promote this gadget as most appropriate for the "modern man," and cordless, battery-powered razors followed the war, along with light-weight plastic models. The twentieth century, then, was mostly a time favoring clean-shaven, short-haired men (plate 15), although the hippie movement among the rebellious youths of the 1960s discouraged any hair management systems at all. As always, hair is manipulated to signal social and political difference.

1. See Will Fisher, "The Renaissance Beard: Masculinity in Early Modern England," *Renaissance Quarterly* 54 (2001): 155–185.

2. From his *Physiologia Barbae Humanae* of 1603, as quoted in Fisher, 174.

3. Pseudo-Aristotle, *Problemata*, as quoted in Zirka Z. Filipczak, *Hot Dry Men/Cold Wet Women* (New York: American Federation of Arts, 1997), 69.

4. Paul Gerbod, *Histoire de la Coiffure et des Coiffeurs* (Paris: Larousse, 1995), 66.

5. Edmundo Desnoes, "'Will You Ever Shave Your Beard?'" in *On Signs*, ed. Marshall Blonsky (Baltimore: Johns Hopkins Press, 1985), 12–13. For Castro, beards signaled commitment to the Revolution.

6. Thomas Stoughton, in his *The Christians Sacrifice* of 1622, as quoted in A. R. Jones and P. Stallybrass, *Renaissance Clothing and the Materials of Memory* (Cambridge: Cambridge University Press, 2000), 79.

7. London, 1628, unpaginated; quotes from the Norwood, N.J.: Walter J. Johnson, 1976 reprint.

8. See M. Dorothy George, *English Political Caricature: A Study of Opinion and Propaganda* (Oxford: Clarendon Press, 1959), I, 24–25.

9. Richard Corson, *Fashions in Hair: The First Five Thousand Years* (London: Peter Owen, 1971), 210–215.

10. Reprinted in John Demos, ed., *Remarkable Providences* (New York: G. Braziller, 1972), 213–220.

11. Marcia Pointon, "The Case of the Dirty Beau: Symmetry, Disorder, and the Politics of Masculinity," in *The Body Imaged*, ed. Kathleen Adler and Marcia Pointon (Cambridge: Cambridge University Press, 1993), 175–189, discusses the wig and masculinity.

12. Massachusetts in 1721 outlawed extravagant wigs. See Corson, *Fashions in Hair*, 262. On American colonial hair styles and attitudes toward wigs, see Wayne Craven, *Colonial American Portraiture* (Cambridge and New York: Cambridge University Press, 1986), especially chapter 3.

13. Bill Severn, *The Long and Short of It: Five Thousand Years of Fun and Fury over Hair* (New York: McKay Co., 1971), 87.

14. On fashions for men's facial hair, see Dwight E. Robinson, "Fashions in Shaving and Trimming of the Beard: The Men of the *Illustrated London News*, 1842–1972," *American Journal of Sociology* 81 (1976), 1133–1141.

15. G. Bruce Retallack, "Razors, Shaving, and Gender Construction: An Inquiry into the Material Culture of Shaving," *Material History Review* 49 (1999): 4.

SEX AND SENSIBILITY: HAIR IN THE MACARONI CARICATURES OF THE 1770S

Amelia Rauser

IN THE EARLY 1770S, a new sort of creature took London by storm: the macaroni. Named for the pasta dish that rich young Grand Tourists brought back from their sojourns in Rome, the macaroni was first known as an elite figure marked by the cultivation of European travel. But as *The Macaroni and Theatrical Magazine* explained in its inaugural issue in 1772, "the word Macaroni then changed its meaning to that of a person who exceeded the ordinary bounds of fashion; and is now justly used as a term of reproach to all ranks of people, indifferently, who fall into this absurdity."[1]

How did a macaroni "exceed the bounds of fashion"? Many aspects of his clothing were extreme, particularly in their exaggerations of scale: tiny shoes were crowned with enormous buckles or rosettes; very tight breeches and vests were worn underneath cutaway coats; fancy sprigged silks were coupled with large, bow-tied cravats.[2] But in the many satirical prints made to represent macaroni men (and women),[3] one feature of the *toilette* especially stands out: their hair. It is in the representation of and reaction to the macaronis' elaborate and oversized hairstyles that we can really see the meaning and import of this strange figure of 1770s culture.

In fact, what was at stake in the amused furor over the macaroni was the proper limit of politeness. As an icon of sophistication who also blurred the boundaries of class and gender, the macaroni was the flashpoint for debates over how the rising middle classes should grapple with their new wealth—how they could properly become urbane sophisticates while remaining authentically British. On one hand, in his adoption of a look that deliberately flaunted artifice, decadence, and the pursuit of pleasure, the macaroni represented an apotheosis of aristocratic values that flew in the face of newer, bourgeois standards for social behavior. On the other hand, the fact that "all ranks of people" were capable of becoming macaronis meant that macaroni-dom was one possible outcome of the modern pursuit of individualism and social mobility central to emergent bourgeois mores. Thus, the macaroni was a "self-made" man, both for good and for ill. Because hair was traditionally associated with sex and power, and the wig with identity play, the macaroni's extravagant hairstyle became the focus both of his challenge to emerging bourgeois manners and of the ridicule that followed him.

This dilemma is at the heart of the 1774 satire *What Is This My Son Tom* (plate 22). In this print, a rustic farmer comes to London and is aghast at the transformation of his son, a country boy, into a macaroni. He pokes with his whip at the tiny hat atop his son's enormous wig, a typical macaroni hairstyle that couples a tall front with a fat "club" of hair hanging down behind. But the viewer is not meant only to laugh at the macaroni and learn from his example. Rather, the print dramatizes a contrast in manners, between too-refined elegance on one hand and too-rough rusticity on the other. The verse beneath the image carefully draws a distinction between true sensibility in dress, which would presumably pass without ridicule, and the modern excess emblematized by the macaroni: "Our wise Forefathers wou'd express/ Ev'n Sensibility in Dress;/ The modern Race delight to Show/ What Folly in Excess can do." But with his coarse posture, straggling hair, and old-fashioned frock coat, the farmer is no exemplar of "sensibility in dress" either. Instead, the lesson in manners is to find the middle way, to cultivate one's sensibility and worldly sophistication while somehow remaining "natural" and authentic. For Britons newly confronted with a wealth of goods and entertainments in a period of booming colonial trade, the question was how to become sophisticated, refined and cosmopolitan, without going overboard into the realm of the laughable, inauthentic macaroni.

In fact, during this macaroni moment the virtue of artifice, as represented by the charged symbolism of the wig, was itself being debated. The illegibility of the macaroni's class and gender made many contemporary theorists of character and manners uncomfortable and caused them to disdain "artificial" manners and to champion instead "sensibility," the expression of politeness based on emotional sensitivity and a passionate heart.[4] This view represented a change. For most of the eighteenth century, artifice was considered a necessary lubricant to social intercourse, smoothing the rough jostling of instinct and will. Further, public life was seen as frankly theatrical, and the wig, which ruled men's fashion only from about 1660 to 1800, made absolutely clear the artificiality of a man's public persona, as part of the costume men put on to assume their proper identity.[5] Wigs were the visible symbol of male authority, styled to reflect the man's age, profession, and social stature (a valence that remains in the term "bigwig").[6] In fact, a 1770 treatise noted that in particular hair "may be dress'd to produce in us different ideas of the qualities of men...who alter their dress according to the different characters they are to perform."[7]

This social meaning of the wig can be seen in William Hogarth's *Midnight Modern Conversation* of 1732 (plate 21), one of the best-loved and most-reproduced prints of the eighteenth century. The debauchery and drunkenness of the group is signified partly by their facial expressions and postures, but their slipped, half-cocked, or altogether missing wigs are the most eloquent clues to the men's overindulgence in punch. While men did sit without their wigs at home and in private (often wearing a cloth cap instead, as does the pipe-smoking man at left in Hogarth's print), the accidental exposure of a man's bald head was held to be acutely embarrassing, akin to a man dropping his pants.

By contrast, women were expected to wear their own hair. During the 1770s, women's hairstyles too reached unprecedented heights; one frequent joke held that because their hair was so tall, ladies were forced to sit on the floors of their carriages in order to fit inside. But complete artifice was disallowed for women's hairstyles. However augmented by false hair, padding, powder, and decorations, women's hairstyles were properly to remain "natural," personal, and distinct from the public and frankly artificial dress of men's hair. Thus, while women's fashionable hair was just as much a topic of critique as men's in the 1770s, the terms of critique were slightly different. The women's fault was in their deceptiveness, their use of fashion and cosmetics to obscure their age and ugliness, and in the lavish expense and moral corruption that following fashion entailed. *Beauty's Lot* (plate 17), for example, emphasizes the ancient vanitas theme, the idea that the material pleasures of this earth are fleeting, and that one should instead concentrate on the health of one's eternal soul. But unlike male fashion victims, the female here is being chastised not for her phoniness or her improper embrace of an inappropriate public role via a large wig (as was the case in *What Is This My Son Tom*), but instead for her vanity and shortsightedness: "As I now am, so You will be."

Because of the social meaning of wigs, then, the extravagantly large wigs worn by macaronis during the early 1770s gave special prominence to their embrace of artifice, theatricality, and identity as play, precisely at the same moment when this artificiality in manners was being questioned and authentic and natural sensibility promoted instead. But here we should pause and consider the status of our evidence. Were "real" macaronis—the men who actually wore tall wigs and tight breeches—as extreme as the fellows in these satires that remain to us today? It seems unlikely. In fact, just as the meaning of the term "macaroni" expanded during the early 1770s, so the image of the macaroni in print and text became more laughable and extreme than the real men whose style and behavior formed the prototype. Furthermore, the earliest macaroni prints, which illustrated named and known macaronis, were much tamer than the later satires that depicted the macaroni as a "type" or generic character.

In fact, caricatural social satire was a relatively new genre which sprang to life in tandem with the macaroni craze, and which shared many of its paradoxical features.[8] Caricature was itself an Italian import; invented in the artistic studios of Baroque Rome, it was, like pasta, brought back to London by aristocratic Grand Tourists as a souvenir of their journey and the wit and cultivation it symbolized.[9] Caricaturing became a favorite parlor game and amusement at country houses among the elite. As the craze for homemade caricatures grew, print publishers Matthew and Mary Darly relocated their shop from Fleet Street, where print sellers were traditionally clustered, to the fashionable West End of London. There, between 1771 and 1773, the Darlys published six sets of satirical "macaroni" prints, each set containing twenty-four portraits, which inspired a whole genre of contemporary social satires. These prints were so popular that the new Darly shop became known (and represented) as "the Macaroni Print-Shop."[10] Other printmakers, like James Sayers and Carington Bowles, soon followed the trend.

The space of the Darlys' print shop reinforced the cultural significance of the macaroni. Beyond treating the joys and dangers of fashion in their subject matter, the macaroni prints were fashionable items in themselves, commodities for sale in a shop that in its location and appointments appealed to an expanding consumer culture in London. In the second half of the eighteenth century, London was rife with new sorts of luxury goods imported from colonies that were enriching Britons at an unprecedented rate. This luxury culture provoked both excitement and anxiety among the swelling ranks of the middle classes, and the figure of the macaroni became their focal point. Thus, the life of the macaroni in print is perhaps even more important than the life of real macaronis, for it was as a symbol that the macaroni was most represented and discussed in the 1770s.

One rich site for examining the symbolism of the macaroni is *The Macaroni and Theatrical Register*, a London journal that lasted for just over a year in 1772–1773, at the height of the macaroni craze. It yoked together the worlds of theater and fashion, featuring short articles reviewing the latest plays in London and tidbits of theatrical gossip.

It also featured a macaroni print to begin each issue, each illustrating an article telling the history of the highlighted, unnamed—but known—macaroni. But besides theater and macaronis, the magazine was filled with essays on behavior, manners, and decorum for both men and women. Articles like "The Character of a Gentleman," "The Art of Being Well-Bred in the Streets," and "An Essay on Politeness" appeared in every issue.

Increasing cultivation was considered a social good, marking high cultural achievement that promised Britain might at last rival France in the cultural arena. "Good breeding is a *social virtue*," the journal proclaimed; "it is benevolence brought into action, with all the advantages and beauty of proportion and symmetry."[11] Further, some essayists argued that manners and up-to-date fashion did not cloak character with artifice, but in some way constituted it. Indeed, one poetic list of gentlemanly traits began not with the man's "inner" qualities, but with his appearance: "A Decent mien, and elegance of dress."[12] But at the same time, other essays and poems in the very same journal demonstrated that readers were petrified of losing something real and authentic as they strove to become more artfully mannered and polite.

This anxiety is discussed in "An Essay on Politeness," published in March 1773: "Modern politeness however which is so ornamental, is very apt to run into disagreeable extremes; amongst the French it is too often disguised by affectation and insincerity…. There must indeed be something very arbitrary in politeness…."[13] The old acceptance of artifice as a necessary part of public life was giving way to a new fear of the deceptiveness, corruption, and arbitrariness of manners. "English courtiers imagine themselves the sole possessors of polite behavior, which they dispense to the Macaronies," but such politeness is as arbitrary as the custom of sneezing among the inhabitants of Monomotapa, claimed the author of "Thoughts on Elegance and Politeness."[14] Despite his high position in society, then, a courtier or macaroni could be considered as strange and unnatural as an isolated islander.

Besides his fluid and illegible class origins, his extravagant dress, and his affected manners, the macaroni was also an icon of artifice because he was linked with the masquerade, as seen in *The Pantheon Macaroni* (plate 20). Once again, the most salient feature of this macaroni is his enormous wig. The Pantheon in London, famed for its masquerade balls, opened right during this macaroni moment, and its elegant public rooms were prime hunting grounds for the macaroni. Party-goers paid a small fee to enter the rooms at the Pantheon dressed either in character costume (as a milkmaid or Henry VIII, for example) or in a domino, the unisex costume comprised of a black silk gown, mask, and tricorn hat.[15] Custom held that all revelers, except royalty, unmasked at midnight. Such balls were seen as places of sexual dalliance and moral depravity, since participants could leave their regular identities behind and masquerade as other classes and even other genders. The masquerade dramatized the thrill and the danger of self-creation, precisely the same issues focused on the macaroni himself.

The sin of artifice and the masquerade is emphasized in *The Modern Paradise; or, Adam and Eve Regenerated*, 1780. This "Modern Paradise" is not an Eden of sexual innocence, free of sin, but rather a landscape filled with all the sinful pleasures of contemporary London. The couple's huge hairstyles signify their immoral and artificial social veneer, as opposed to the state of nature represented by their nude bodies. But the size and extravagance of their hair also signals the amount of corruption they've mastered—so much that they've outdone the devil, who is on his way back to Hell. The "tree of life" in this Eden is marked by the names of new gambling houses and clubs, and by the Pantheon. The serpent between the man's legs and the "lap dog" climbing up the lady's allude to their decadent sexuality. "Implements for procuring heirs to estates," at the feet of the lady, include a masquerade ticket and a mask (referring to the adulterous sex that took place at masquerades), while the "Implements for saddling an estate"—with debt, that is—are a jockey's hat, saddle, and whip, the tools for gambling and frittering away the family wealth on the horses. Meanwhile, in the background, "Cain and Abel" duel. Thrift, hard work, chastity, piety, family—all these bourgeois virtues are mocked and subverted by this decadent couple whose macaroni hairstyles epitomize their decadence.

Another key feature of his challenge to emergent bourgeois norms was the macaroni's curious sexuality. Like his artifice, it too was emblematized by his enormous hairstyle. Hair's ancient association with sexuality was heightened in the eighteenth century, which was also the heyday of the merkin, or pubic wig. Extreme macaroni hair represented a particularly potent or depraved version of sexuality, and was seen in satires of both male and female fashion victims. Among the many "hairstyle satires" Matthew and Mary Darly published in the 1770s was *Oh-Heigh-Oh; or, A View of the Back Settlements* (plate 18). In an era when women's fanciest hairstyles functioned as theatrical set pieces, even in one case supposedly staging the battle of Bunker Hill, this print combines fashion satire with political valences, referring in the name ("Ohio") to the subject on every Londoner's lips in the summer of 1776, the American Colonies. But the imagery and the coy subtitle are overtly sexual. The woman's hairstyle is framed by a lace-edged bonnet that appears like an upswept petticoat. Underneath, her fat curls are arranged into a visual analog of female genitalia, with a flirty ostrich plume pointing suggestively towards them.

But the relationship between extreme hair and sexuality was not straightforward. *The Enrag'd Macaroni*, 1773, also analogizes wig and genitalia, but in this case the macaroni is viewed as lacking in manliness. Here, a dandy is "castrated" by having the queue of his wig lopped off by a mischievous woman leaning out of a gin shop; he himself echoes this action by unsheathing his knife in a dangerous position. The altercation between dandy and fishwife on the streets of London was actually an established genre; examples generally paired feisty female street vendors against foppish and terrified French aristocrats, and showed the women getting the better of them.[16] This updated macaroni version substitutes the homegrown dandy for the wimpy Frenchman, but the charge of sexual weakness and effeminacy remains the same.

Several historians have hazarded that the macaroni might represent an early homosexual subculture.[17] Like the *Enrag'd Macaroni*, the *Pantheon Macaroni*, with his mirrored dressing table, pots of cosmetics, and corsage, certainly seems intended to be read as "effeminate." Further, the cat carved into the chair behind him may provide specific evidence for the claim that the macaroni was associated with homosexual practices; it might be included to mark the man as a "catamite," a young male lover of an older man.[18] But as Shearer West and Philip Carter have argued, such indications of non-standard gender or sexuality must be understood in their eighteenth-century contexts, and not as they would be read today.[19] Contemporaries often explained the macaroni as too narcissistic, too eccentric, or simply too physically weak to be properly sexual, rather than as homosexual. Textual commentary on the macaroni often characterized him as a "hermaphrodite" or "amphibious creature," or as "The Macaroni; A New Song" put it in 1772: "His taper waist, so strait and long,/ His spindle shanks, like pitchfork prong,/ To what sex does the thing belong?/ 'Tis call'd a Macaroni."[20] Like his class, the macaroni's sex was often illegible.

Indeed, the macaroni was not simply unmanly; instead, his sexuality was both confusing and potentially voracious, and again his hair was his potent sexual symbol. *The Macaroni and Theatrical Magazine* reported in May 1773 an encounter at the Pantheon masquerade between a Lord "dressed as a macaroni buck" and another unnamed nobleman "in the character of a Gardener." The "macaroni" is described solely in terms of his enormous wig: "The club of hair, which was supposed to have proceeded from the Nobleman's head, was of such a prodigious size, that it covered both his shoulders, and was, at a moderate computation, nearly the size of a two-gallon bottle." Contemplating this, the "gardener" is reported to have remarked, "I was thinking what a nice method of wooing you fine folks have got into—you may do it all in dumb shew—and what a world of vexation and trouble it would have saved me, if I had been acquainted with it before I courted my Jannet. But may I ask you a civil question Sir—

for I have woundy curiosity to know—have you not said too much?—is it not larger than the reality?"[21] The analogy between large wig and large genitalia here is humorously undercut by the suggestion of masculine overcompensation.

The macaroni was fascinating to his contemporaries in the 1770s because he represented a last gasp of aristocratic fashionability, decadence, and gender-bending. This was the last decade during which men wore the kind of extravagant, colorful costumes and luxurious fabrics that would thereafter only be acceptable for women. It was also the final hurrah of the wig. Even before revolution broke out in France, men were discarding the wig, as newer values of naturalism and individualism triumphed over old-regime ideals of social artifice and identity play. Only ten years later, with the world transformed by political and social revolution and gender roles hardened, the very idea of the macaroni was beyond the pale. Yet during this decade of tumult and change, the macaroni served a useful purpose in satires and caricature, representing the undesirable extreme of the civilizing process, educating Britons about the limits of eccentricity, and flattering those viewers who were wise enough not to fall, as he did, into the traps of a decadent and luxurious society.[22]

1. *The Macaroni and Theatrical Magazine*, London, October 1772, 1.

2. See Valerie Steele, "The Social and Political Significance of Macaroni Fashion," *Costume* 19 (1985): 94–109.

3. Although the macaronis were initially all male, as the term broadened it occasionally came to include women who were, like their male counterparts, highly fashionable and distinguished by extremely large hairstyles. But it was the male who was the archetypal macaroni, partly because male effeminacy was a crucial part of the macaroni mystique, and partly because it was nothing new for women to be disparaged as vain, decadent, and overly concerned with fashion. In this essay, I will mostly refer to the macaroni as "he."

4. Philip Carter's *Men and the Emergence of Polite Society, Britain 1660–1800* (New York and London: Longman, 2001) is a superb discussion of the role and meaning of sensibility in male identity in this period.

5. Wigs became standard polite dress in England in the 1660s, introduced to the court by Charles II. Paradoxically,

at the same moment Charles instituted a dress reform movement that simplified men's clothing and introduced the earliest version of the three-piece suit.

6. For a good discussion of the significance of wigs in the eighteenth century, see Marcia Pointon, *Hanging the Head* (New Haven and London: Yale University Press, 1993), 114–123.

7. D. Ritchie, *A Treatise on the Hair* (London, 1770), 78, cited by Marcia Pointon, *Hanging the Head*, 107.

8. It is not mere coincidence that social caricature and the macaroni appeared at the same moment in the early 1770s; I believe both are indicators of a systemic crisis in representation of the individual in British society.

9. The best contemporary account of the history of caricature in this period is Diana Donald, *The Age of Caricature: Satirical Prints in the Reign of George III* (New Haven and London: Yale University Press, 1996).

10. See Timothy Clayton, *The English Print*, 1688–1802 (New Haven and London: Yale University Press, 1997), for detailed accounts of printmakers and the print market in eighteenth-century London.

11. "The Character of a Well-Bred Man," *The Macaroni and Theatrical Magazine*, December 1772, 100.

12. From the doggerel ode, "A Character of A Gentleman. Addressed to a Friend," *The Macaroni and Theatrical Magazine*, December 1772, 133. Only later did the poem address qualities that today we might think of as being part of "character," such as his reason, principles, or elevated mind.

13. *The Macaroni and Theatrical Magazine*, March 1773, 264.

14. *The Macaroni and Theatrical Magazine*, August 1773, 492–493.

15. Many excellent accounts of the masquerade exist. For a brief analysis of a real masquerade ball, see Aileen Ribeiro, "The King of Denmark's Masquerade," *History Today* 27, no. 6 (June 1977): 385–389; for a more wide-ranging and theorized account, see Terry Castle, *Masquerade and Civilization: The Carnivalesque in 18th-Century English Culture and Fiction* (Stanford, Calif.: Stanford University Press, 1986).

16. See, for example, *Sal Dab Giving Monsieur a Receipt in Full* of 1766, British Museum catalogue 4623, and *The Frenchman at Market* of 1770, British Museum catalogue 4476.

17. See for example Peter McNeil, "'That Doubtful Gender': Macaroni Dress and Male Sexualities," *Fashion Theory* 3, issue 4 (1999): 411–448.

18. The observation and interpretation of this detail comes from Peter McNeil, "'That Doubtful Gender,'" 426. "Catamite" is a Latinate form of "Ganymede."

19. See Shearer West, "The Darly Macaroni Prints and the Politics of 'Private Man,'" *Eighteenth-Century Life* 25 (Spring 2001): 170–182, and Philip Carter, *Men and the Emergence of Polite Society*.

20. *The Macaroni and Theatrical Magazine*, October 1772, n.p.

21. *The Macaroni and Theatrical Magazine*, May 1773, 372.

22. Philip Carter, *Men and Emergence of Polite Society*, 156.

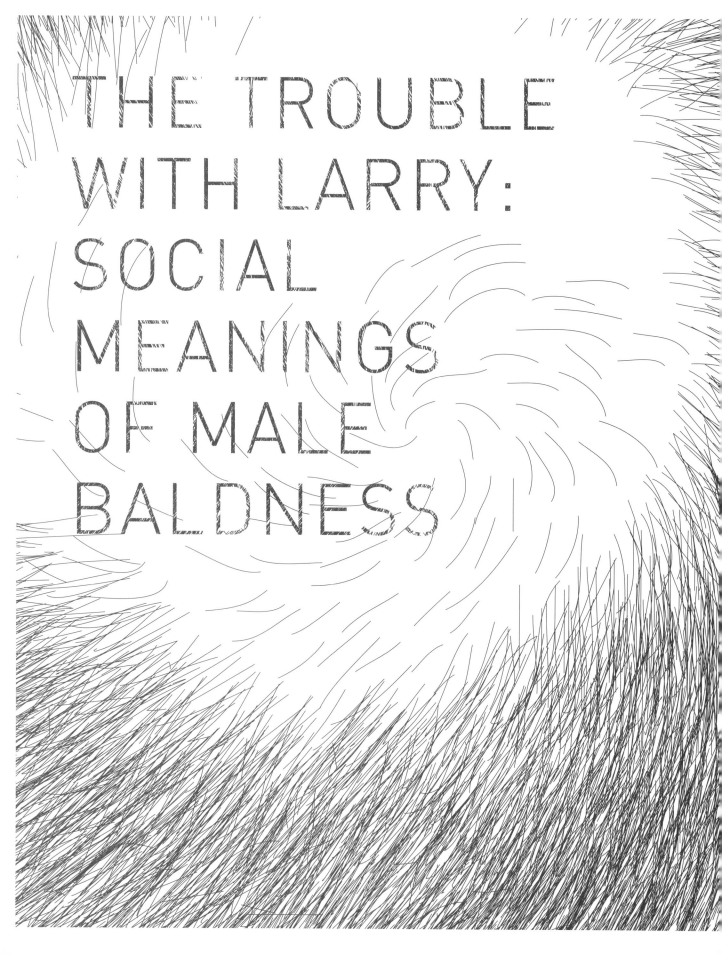

THE TROUBLE WITH LARRY: SOCIAL MEANINGS OF MALE BALDNESS

Susan Walzer

"BALD MEN LOVE OTHER BALD MEN," Larry David writes. "There's a bonding that takes place on some deep level that you never get with anyone else. We've been through it. We live with it."[1] What is the "it" with which bald men live? One answer to this question is that the experiences of bald men are influenced by a long-standing socially constructed equation of hair loss with powerlessness and undermining of masculinity. The "it" with which bald men live is the unfortunate human tendency to use physical characteristics to mark social positions and produce hierarchy. We do it with skin color; we do it with genitals; we do it with what's on top of our heads. And when it comes to domes, for most of history, the "hair guy" has been perceived as having something more than the bald man, and not just hair.

In this essay, I call on current research about impressions and consequences of baldness as well as reviews of attitudes about hair and hairlessness over time to explore the social meanings of baldness.[2] Along with personal narratives, the resources on which I draw reflect the work primarily of dermatologists and psychologists—clinicians motivated perhaps by their occupational encounters with people who are troubled by baldness: both outside and inside of their heads. One article, for example, examines the promotion of medications for "personal and social problems," beginning a list of examples with "male pattern baldness" that also includes "mental fatigue, small breasts, tension, stress, and obesity."[3] This cataloguing of "problems" is instructive in its identification of socially constructed gender violations—small breasts in women and baldness in men. This is the "it" with which bald men live—a long-standing societal view that youthful, powerful, "real" men have hair on their heads.

In a literature review of research about the psychosocial consequences of hair loss (or androgenetic alopecia, as the doctors call it), Thomas Cash reluctantly and qualifiedly summarizes the findings as supporting the notion that visible hair loss has a negative effect on social perceptions.[4] Cash's own experimental work ("losing hair, losing points?") reveals that subjects perceive bald men as older and less attractive than men with hair,[5] although other studies suggest that men may hold these perceptions even more strongly than women,[6] and that bald men may be overly sensitive to other people's reactions.[7]

But that's the problem: hair loss is implicated in low self-esteem and other psychological problems of individuals who experience it.[8] Cash cites a representative survey of more than 1,700 men in four European countries in which hair loss is associated with more worry, helplessness, self-consciousness, and social stress.[9] On the other hand, not all men are troubled by hair loss to the same degree. They feel worse when it happens earlier, when they are romantically unattached, when they're highly self-conscious and invested in their appearance, and when they have lower levels of self-acceptance in general.[10] In other words, baldness may be a hook on which a troubled man hangs his hat. Lest we blame the victim, however, we have to acknowledge the evidence that negative responses to baldness do, in fact, exist.

Many people perceive hair to communicate something in and of itself. In this view, hair is not a reflection of the person; it reflects *on* the person. One study finds, for example, that "bad hair days" have the power to decrease self-esteem, bring out social insecurities, and cause people to be more aware of other flaws besides their "bad" hair.[11] In order to understand the meanings ascribed to baldness, therefore, we have to understand the symbolic importance of hair—to recognize the association of "good" hair with health, youth, and virility.

Across cultures for centuries, Cash writes, hair has been "a medium of social communication and a display of social identity or status."[12] Intrigue with hair and hair loss dates as far back as the forty-century-old medical papyri of the Egyptians. The "physician of the head" was one of the oldest medical specialists, according to Herodotus (484–425 b.c.), and treatments of diseases of the scalp were often accompanied by exorcisms.[13] Giacometti argues that the exposed scalp has historically been considered a "sign of degradation" and makes the dramatic suggestion that the deep-seated mythology associated with the scalp and hair "reflects some underlying, unconscious anxiety which is an inherent biological attribute of the entire race."[14]

Could worry about hair be innate? Giacometti isn't alone in suggesting some biological basis for it. Kligman and Freeman, while noting that "rigorous studies are lacking," nevertheless suggest that bald people may die earlier. They cite a chief surgeon who observed that when Napoleon's army of 500,000 marched into Russia in 1812, retreating with 40,000 survivors, "the bald had died first." As supplementary evidence, they speculate that the reason baldness "increases steadily in white men until about the middle of the sixth decade, and thereafter falls off slightly," is that bald people die earlier than other people.[15]

Hair is associated with youth and brawn while baldness carries associations with aging and deterioration. Monks and priests shave their heads as acts of submission, and the biblical story of Samson and Delilah implies "that a man's loss of hair erodes his masculine strength."[16] Hair is central to women's social position as well. Rose Weitz argues that women use physical attractiveness, and their hair in particular, as a source of power.[17] Women who lose their hair are not just without a source of potency, but may feel abnormal as women—a possible explanation for research findings that hair loss can be even more impairing for women than for men.[18]

Hair loss in men has historically (and in this essay) been given greater attention, however, perhaps because balding leads to men's "complete denudation"[19] and the more specific association of hairiness with masculine domination. The trouble that Larry David identifies is that "hair guys" reign supreme in the social hierarchy and are not threatened by bald men: "We're jokes to them. We're not taken seriously. If a hair guy has a girlfriend, he's never threatened by a bald man. He doesn't mind if his girlfriend has a platonic bald man in her life. He's not worried. 'Come on in, bald man, make yourself at home.' Nothing ever gave me more pleasure than the time I took a woman away from a hair guy." David concludes his analysis with the admittedly self-serving theory that bald men are better lovers. First, because of the appreciation factor: "The bald man is so thrilled to actually be in bed with a woman that he'll do anything and everything, and all with tremendous gusto." And of course, he says, there's the testosterone: "We've got it in spades. That's why we went bald in the first place."[20]

What makes David's commentary especially subversive is that he claims a kind of hypermasculinity and superiority for bald men that goes against centuries of social constructions. For Larry David to be proud of being a bald man "who's out there"—to claim that bald men have more male hormones than hair guys—is to challenge the notion that hair makes the man; or rather, that baldness makes him less of a man. David is apparently not the first to go down this road. Kligman and Freeman cite Aristotle (who just happened to be bald) as suggesting that hair is nurtured by a "mysterious secretion which in libidinous men is dissipated too rapidly"—in other words, baldness is a price men pay for sexual excess.[21]

More recent analyses suggest, however, that balding is a process more powerful than any man's behavior, including the comb-over. And while balding cannot be pre-
vented (except perhaps by castration, as *New York Times* health columnist Jane Brody
asserts),[22] people with head hair are in possession of a body part over which they have
some control. Hair can be manipulated to communicate particular messages, especially by not grooming it in socially expected ways. When people do this with their own
hair, they may feel empowered. Yet when people's hair is cut off by others (as anyone
who has been to an autocratic hairdresser can attest), or by an institution, they are sin-
gularly not in control. In the contexts of the military, imprisonment, or war, the shaving
of hair reflects a "removal of individuality and subjugation to authority."[23] And as
Giacometti writes, "Scalping has long been a custom of cultural significance, the visible proof of personal bravery, the palpable sign of accomplished revenge, the honorable
plunder in battle."[24]

Perhaps this is what makes men with toupees so vulnerable to humiliation:
their scalps are so much easier to take. The final visual blow in the brutal murder of the
despicable Ralphie on television's *Sopranos* was the slipping off of his toupee. Vince
Staten notes that when actor Burt Reynolds filed for bankruptcy in 1996, "he suffered
the embarrassment of having to list debts to two toupee companies, including a whop-
ping $121,796.62 owed to Edward Katz Hair Design."[25]

Unfortunately for Reynolds, there have been other historical eras more con-
ducive to wearing a wig than our own. Although the impulse to correct baldness does
go back as far as the ancient Egyptians, wigs have not always been used just as a cover,
but also as a fashion accessory to enhance one's attractiveness.[26] In our time, however, the man who chooses to cover his baldness is apparently in a no-win situation, his
very solution a potential arena for ridicule.

Larry David is contemptuous of all attempts by bald men to distract from or
cover baldness. David presents the scenario of a bald man with a baseball cap meeting a woman in the park. The meeting leads to a date and now the bald man has a
"dilemma." Addressing the bald man, David chides: "You made your first mistake by
going out with the hat. You think she's going to like it when you show up at her door with
your chrome? What she's going to be is disappointed that you misrepresented yourself.
You've tried to come off as a hair guy. You've lied, bald man."[27]

The theme of authenticity also comes up in Vince Staten's commentary about
his own flirtation with a toupee: "I was simply trying to pretend I wasn't bald. And you
can't do that. If you are bald, you are bald and no fancy piece of fabric and fluff can

alter that." Staten refers to the toupee as a "cover-up and nothing more." But with a subtext of ambivalence he goes on to say that part of his decision to forego the toupee was that he knew he couldn't "fool" everyone; "there were too many people who knew me as a baldie—so I would be living a lie."[28]

We do have a tendency to find cover-ups worse than crimes, but there may be no better time in history to be an openly bald man, especially one who looks like he is doing it on purpose. While the appeal of actors Telly Savalas and Sean Connery hasn't hurt the white man, it is the iconic African-American basketball player, Michael Jordan, who has popularized hairless pates. His shaved bald head, as Jeffrey Segrave notes, has made "the phallic look chic among millions of young men around the world."[29]

Jordan's legitimization of the hairless head is not without social and political implications, however. As Ingrid Banks argues, we use hair in our culture not just for gender, but for racial classification. Her study of African-American women suggests that social definitions of "good" hair can be a way of maintaining racial hierarchy. People of color may respond to dominant definitions of "good" (read "white") hair either by trying to get it, thus maintaining the status quo, or by leaning into their difference and thereby subverting the status quo.[30] When Michael Jordan shaves his head and removes one of the visible symbols of African-American identity, Segrave argues, he distracts from another part of him that is even more politically relevant and intractable: his black skin. Elevating a behavior that some have argued is just another unsuccessful attempt to cure baldness,[31] Michael Jordan, at the same time, neutralizes his difference and enhances his ability to sell himself and numerous products in the capitalist economy.[32]

If there's profit in undoing differences, it follows that bald people remain vulnerable to the commodification of "cures" for their condition. Two "authorities" on hair style, writing in 1970, predicted that by the year 2001, through the use of color sprays and wigs, "baldness will be obsolete. Men will no longer accept baldness as a natural state of affairs."[33] Although their prophecy of the disappearance of baldness has not come to pass, the point that people will try to intervene in it (and the implicit suggestion that other people will make money doing so) is certainly accurate. As Adele Ferguson writes, current options vary from "basic to esoteric"—from toupees (known in the hair industry as "units") to electronic treatments, hair transplants, and lateral scalp reductions in which "strips of skin are removed and hairlines are pulled back together using staples and stitches."[34] A website I saw reported that in 2001 the sales of hair-growth product Rogaine totalled $117 million.

Moerman likens the clinical condition of androgenetic alopecia to other kinds

43

of "communication disorders" such as stuttering and lisping, and suggests that it is not a surprise that people would seek treatment. Like people with speech disorders, Moerman writes, bald men "are communicating something they may not wish to convey," simply by being bald.[35] People with hair on their heads, on the other hand, can voluntarily use it to communicate anything they'd like. One young man commented in an interview, for example, that "being a white kid in a white kid school," it made him more distinctive to other people to dye his hair.[36] Larry David would argue, however, that this is a privilege of hair guys, who have more choice than bald men about how other people interpret their heads.

To conclude on an optimistic note, maybe people do not always form their impressions only by the state of the pate. One can take comfort, as Adele Ferguson writes, in "all the historic figures not remembered [primarily, I would add] for being bald: Winston Churchill, William Shakespeare, Pablo Picasso, and Queen Elizabeth I."[37] In the end, baldness, like sex or race, becomes a physical characteristic best addressed with self-acceptance as well as a critique of the use of physical differences to mark social positions and maintain power hierarchies. Even though human beings categorize, stereotype, and oppress each other, we also have the capacity to decide not to. Want to commit a tiny revolutionary act? Let go of being troubled by baldness.

1. Larry David, "Kiss My Head," *Men's Fashions of the Times Magazine*, 19 March 2001, 108.

2. For research assistance on this topic, I am indebted to Elizabeth Umbro and Michelle Blocklin, with whom I presented an earlier version of this paper at the 2002 Skidmore College Senior Symposium.

3. Michael Montagne, "The Promotion of Medications for Personal and Social Problems," *Journal of Drug Issues* 22 (1992): 389–405.

4. Thomas F. Cash, "The Psychological Consequences of Androgenetic Alopecia: A Review of the Research Literature," *British Journal of Dermatology* 141 (1999): 398–405.

5. Thomas F. Cash, "Losing Hair, Losing Points? The Effects of Male Pattern Baldness on Social Impression Formation," *Journal of Applied Social Psychology* 20 (1990): 154–167.

6. Daniel E. Moerman, "The Meaning of Baldness and Implications for Treatment," *Clinics in Dermatology* 6 (1988): 89–92.

7. Michael S. Wogalter and Judith A. Hosie, "Effects of Cranial and Facial Hair on Perceptions of Age and Person," *Journal of Social Psychology* 131 (1991): 589–591.

8. See Cash, "Psychological Consequences," as well as E. B. G. DeKoning, J. Passchier, and F.W. Dekker, "Psychological Problems with Hair Loss in General Practice and the Treatment of General Practitioners," *Psychological Reports* 67 (1990): 775–778, and J. Passchier, S. E. Rijpma, R. O. G .M. Dutrée-Meulenberg, F. Verhage, and E. Stolz, "Why Men with Hair Loss Go to the Doctor," *Psychological Reports* 65 (1989): 323–330.

9. See study by D. Budd et al., 1997, cited in Cash, "Psychological Consequences."

10. Cash, "Psychological Consequences."

11. Marianne LaFrance, "An Experimental Investigation into the Effects of 'Bad Hair,'" unpublished study

conducted for Proctor and Gamble's *Physique* Hair Care Line (2000): 1–44.

12. See Cash, "Psychological Consequences," 398.

13. Luigi Giacometti, "Facts, Legends, and Myths about the Scalp throughout History," *Archives of Dermatology* 95 (1967): 629–631.

14. Giacometti, "Facts, Legends, and Myths," 631.

15. Albert M. Kligman and Beth Freeman, "History of Baldness: From Magic to Medicine," *Clinical Dermatology* 6 (1988): 85.

16. Cash, "Psychological Consequences," 398.

17. Rose Weitz, "Women and Their Hair: Seeking Power through Resistance and Accommodation," *Gender and Society* 15 (2001): 667–686.

18. Cash, "Psychological Consequences."

19. Kligman and Freeman, "History of Baldness," 84.

20. David, "Kiss My Head," 108.

21. Kligman and Freeman, "History of Baldness," 84.

22. Brody is cited in Richard Liebmann-Smith's article, "Bald is Beautiful," in *Utne Reader* 106 (July/August 2001): 45.

23. Cash, "Psychological Consequences," 398.

24. Giacometti, "Facts, Legends, and Myths," 630.

25. Vince Staten, *Do Bald Men Get Half-Price Haircuts? In Search of America's Great Barbershops* (New York: Touchstone, 201), 126.

26. William Andrews, *At the Sign of the Barber's Pole: Studies in Hirsute History* (Cottingham, Yorkshire: J. R. Tutin, 1904).

27. David, "Kiss My Head," 108.

28. Staten, *Do Bald Men Get Half-Price Haircuts?* 128. The circumstances under which one gets away with covering baldness may include spending a million dollars to do so, which Adele Ferguson, in "Of Follicles, Fallacies, and Fads," *Business Review Weekly* 19 (1997): 92–93, writes is the amount Elton John is reported to have spent on his hair transplant.

29. Jeffrey O. Segrave, "(H)Air Jordan: Excavating His Royal Baldness," this volume, 78.

30. Ingrid Banks, *Hair Matters: Beauty, Power, and Black Women's Consciousness* (New York: New York University Press, 2000).

31. Tom Junod, "Hair Apparent," *Esquire* 129 (1998): 20.

32. Segrave, "(H)Air Jordan."

33. Ann Charles and Roger DeAnfrasio, *The History of Hair: An Illustrated Review of Hair Fashions for Men Throughout the Ages* (New York: Bonanza Books, 1970), 213.

34. Adele Ferguson, "Of Follicles, Fallacies, and Fads," 92–93.

35. Moerman, "Meaning of Baldness," 92.

36. Michelle Blocklin and Susan Walzer, "It's about Control: Toward a Sociology of Hair," presentation at the 2002 Skidmore College Senior Week Symposium.

37. Ferguson, "Follicles, Fallacies, and Fads," 93.

THE IDEAL
WOMAN

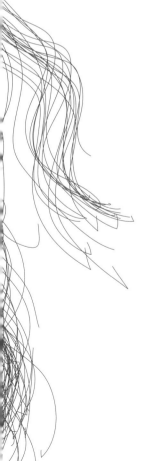

Penny Howell Jolly

TWO IDEALS CONCERNING WOMEN'S HAIR have had remarkable longevity in western society: it should be long and its color should be blonde.

With regard to length, women's hair—with rare exception, as noted below—was understood to be "naturally" long; however, it was still to be appropriately controlled in accordance with social codes. For example, in fifteenth-century Europe, young unmarried women wore their hair long and flowing, a signal of their sexuality but also of their virginity—the appropriate state for the prospective bride; instead of today's symbolic white gown, brides in wedding images symbolically wear their hair down. Once actually married, European women wore their hair fastened up on their heads, sometimes in elaborate braids and interwoven with pearls and ribbons, as in Florence, or, in Flemish cities, in paired horns called *cornes*.[1] Like the modern wedding band, these hair styles marked the woman as unavailable to suitors. Pearls signaled chastity, as did the decorous binding of the hair: often even ears were chastely covered by a cap or braid, because of the belief that Mary conceived Christ through her ear.[2] Veils or other coverings protected the wife's hair from public view. Her hair would be unbound in private, signaling her openness to her husband; movies today still use a woman's letting down of her hair as a signal of sexual surrender. In addition to hair pulled up away from the face, plucked hairlines and eyebrows accentuated a smooth, rounded forehead.

Thus Renaissance images of the Virgin Mary, where she is frequently shown with long, flowing hair, even in public settings, immediately signaled her status as both

Virgin and Bride of Christ. Modern viewers of the long-haired Mary holding or even nursing the infant Christ might simply see her hair as a mark of her youthfulness and femininity. To Renaissance viewers, however, her hair was socially and theologically significant. By symbolizing her virginal state, her hair reminded viewers of the miraculous nature of the Incarnation: a Virgin has given birth. Thus the wonder of the divine event was enhanced by the wonderfully contradictory message of her hair: here is an untouched Virgin mother who nurtures her child.

Italian Renaissance writers also established the blonde as the perfect female, her fairness expressive of innocence and purity. Of course this was a difficult ideal for predominantly dark-haired Italian women to attain.[3] Even today in our country, with its wide-reaching ethnic mix, no more than 17 percent of women are natural blondes.[4] Following the lead from classical and medieval sources favoring blondeness, the fourteenth-century poet Petrarch expressed the preference for fair hair that prevails through much of modern western tradition. Praising his beloved Laura, he writes of "Those tresses of gold, which ought to make the sun go filled with envy," and how "Amid the locks of gold Love hid the noose with which he bound me."[5] In his *Dialogue on the Beauty of Women* of 1548, Agnolo Firenzuola has his protagonist, Celso, state: "You know that the proper and true color of hair should be blonde."[6] How did Italian women respond? Like their classical sisters before them, they turned to bleaching and dyeing processes; to powdering hair with pollen or even gold dust; to applying lemon juice and saffron concoctions, and spreading hair out over wide-brimmed, crownless straw hats to dry in the sun, as courtesans in Venice did; or to wearing wigs made of northern Europeans' hair. Processes could be dangerous or unpleasant—both lye and horse urine were sometimes used—as Giovanni Marinelli warns in his censorious *On the Adornments of Women* of 1562.[7] Churchmen, of course, decried the vanity and deceptive unnaturalness of such doings; monk and reformer Savonarola burned wigs in his bonfires of the vanities in Florence as early as the 1490s, and in 1585 Philip Stubbes, who calls dyed hair an "ornament of pride," complains of people manipulating children into selling their "faire haire."[8] As is often the case, fashion and religion were at odds.

Artists also helped to promote blondeness, as many a Renaissance Italian portrait shows an ideally beautiful woman, but perhaps with deceptively blonde hair. In all time periods, images can represent imaginary ideals or symbolic ideas rather than mirror true practice. Sixteenth-century Venice particularly celebrated the blonde, as documented in countless images by Titian and his followers; probably these women would be unrecognizable in real life as compared to their portraits. The ideal extends to narrative imagery as well, as in Paolo Veronese's *Rebecca at the Well* from circa 1570–1580 (plate 23). Even though Veronese depicts an Old Testament scene where Rebecca is chosen as wife for Isaac while drawing water from the well, he represents this Hebrew beauty as a sixteenth-century blonde in Venetian finery. She wears her golden hair raised and curled upon her head, as all Veronese's heroic females do. By contrast, red hair was reserved for evil figures, especially Jews. Judas was supposedly a redhead, as was Cain, the first murderer, and Jacob's "ruddy" and hirsute brother, Esau.

Sixteenth-century Europe included a number of developments regarding hair. In 1545, the first metal hairpins were used in England, and by the later sixteenth century, changing fashion encouraged women to supplement their natural hair by combing it over pads or wire frames.[9] Wigs also returned briefly, after centuries of being out of fashion. Although popular in ancient cultures, not until the late sixteenth-century court of Elizabeth I did highborn women turn to wigs, especially blonde ones. Once the Queen's natural reddish-blonde hair began to gray and thin, she acquired as many as eighty wigs to maintain an appearance of perpetual youth and virginity. At her court, wig snatching became a crime.[10]

The seventeenth century ushered in a number of changes with regard to women's hair, as blonde went out of fashion in favor of dark hair with elaborate ringlets and curls; again, it was the French court, especially Louis XIV's, that established the new fashion, and stylish women in England and elsewhere followed suit. By contrast, women in Protestant Holland wore their hair held tightly to their scalps and covered by a small cap; fashions were similarly less elaborate in the New World colonies. This was also a time when wigs were more important to men—who routinely wore them to create their long, fashionable styles—than to women, although females certainly used false curls and smaller hairpieces, especially for the more elaborate "tower" styles of the late century, where one's hair and false curls were arranged over a wire foundation.

But it was in the 1750s through 1770s that hair styles became perhaps their most extravagant, and wigs became common on upper-class European women. Unfortunately, the pomades used to help shape and hold their hair constructions were typically lard-based, and the powder was edible flour. There are not only tales of mice, lice, and other vermin living in these greased and floured "nests" of hair, but also descriptions of various ornaments attached to the elaborate erections, such as ships, wagons, flowers set in bottles of water to remain fresh, and even glow worms.[11] Thus, to improve hygiene most cut their natural hair short and resorted to wigs, leaving some hair as a base for attaching the heavy devices. These pretentious styles encouraged the biting satires published in England in the later eighteenth century, mocking the French-inspired hairdos and customs of upper-class women and men. The 1780 English etching of *The Modern Paradise, or Adam and Eve Regenerated* depicts the first couple wearing outrageously large powdered hairdos, Eve's even including feathers and horns. The anonymous writer refers to them as "Sir and Madam" and assures the reader these "Modern Adams and Eves" are so "Improved in each Vice and each Folly that's going…That They capable seem to impose on the Devil."[12] Hunters shoot at birds and animals that unknowingly nest in women's elaborately towering hair artifices, mistaking them for trees (plate 19), while other women crouch down on the floors of carriages, the seats having been removed so they can actually fit inside without crushing their high coiffures. Actual accounts reveal that hair structures could be as tall as three feet, and so some were partially removable, allowing women to travel to social affairs, where the hair could be restored before entering.

Of course, the aristocratic fashion for elaborate, powdered hair did not survive the French Revolution, for women as well as men by the 1790s determined to express their political ideologies via dress and specifically by changing to less contrived and unpowdered hair styles.[13] Like men, women adopted the Titus hair cut and generally simplified their *toilettes* in a return to what was seen as a more natural and austere fashion, one suggestive of youth, purity, and innocence. We see a fine example of this "republican" style, now transplanted to the newly formed United States—also a post-revolutionary context—in James Peale's *Portrait of Jane Ramsey Peale* from about 1802 (plate 25). Not only is her make-up simplified in comparison to earlier aristocratic styles and her white muslin dress of the new high-waisted, low-cut bodice style, based on Greco-Roman precedents, but shorter hair frames her face in light unpowdered ringlets, the whole held together by a casually tied head scarf. Although conceived within an ideology of *liberté, égalité, et fraternité*, the revolutionary dress and hair style quickly became fashionable, and was emulated by the rising high society of early nineteenth-century Europe and America.

Early nineteenth-century fashion celebrated a return to natural hair color, and thus being a brunette—the most common hair color for humans in nature—became fashionable throughout much of the century in western culture: it was in 1854 that Stephen Foster wrote his famous "I Dream of Jeanie with the Light Brown Hair." But while brunette remained the preferred color, men quickly complained regarding the lack of femininity in the new century's short styles, and professional hairdressers protested that the simple hairdos were driving them out of work. What began in the 1810s as simple topknots developed, in the 1820s and 1830s, into elaborate mounds of hair with loops and curls, knobs that imitated those of giraffes, and flowers and ribbons (plate 26). Hairdressers were back in business, as long hair returned to style, and false curls and hairpieces were once again displayed in fashion books as necessary for women. While fashion continued to change dramatically in mid-century, to hair that was low and sleek on the crown and typically parted in the middle, curls and braids were still added, but now to the backs and/or sides, often covering the ears.

Examples of such fashions are found in the *Godey's Lady's Book*, a monthly fashion, housekeeping, craft, and general advice magazine for women, begun in 1830 and calling itself "America's first magazine."[14] It claimed to bring the newest of French fashion to this country, for Paris was still the fashion capital. Although Edgar Allan Poe's *Graham's American Monthly Magazine of Literature, Art and Fashion* had in fact preceded it by almost four years, *Godey's* did remain the most popular American fashion publication of the century. Each month, a hand-colored plate displayed the latest in dress, accessories, and hair styles, for both women and children. Already in the sixteenth century, fashion plates were printed to circulate contemporary fashions. But by the mid-nineteenth century, more than one hundred fashion periodicals were in publication in Europe alone; in this country, eighteen women's magazines were produced in the 1880s. The *Godey's* illustrations, seen by 150,000 subscribers across the nation, offered women up-to-date styling for their dress and their hair—including suggestions for clustering curled ringlets at the nape of the neck and looping multi-colored ribbons through the hair.

The market for hair products and artificial hair, including chignons, ringlets, and curls, boomed during the nineteenth century, with major hair traders and marketers centered in Paris. In 1856, 11,954 chignons were exported from France to England, while in 1862, approximately one hundred tons of hair was sold, with French and Italian hair most desirable, and white or gray hair the most expensive.[15] In 1859–1860 in the United States, 200,000 pounds of hair was imported for the making of hairpieces.[16] Throughout this time period brunette hair remained favored, and dyes proliferated, along with pomades, ointments, hair restorers, and tonics: of course dark hair colors were easier to obtain than light, and dark brown and black dyes were most popular. For women, luxuriant length was greatly prized, as seen in advertisements in this exhibition for hair care products featuring women such as Martha Matilda Harper (1857–1950)—an enterprising hair tonic and shampoo producer and beauty salon owner who began marketing her products in 1888 and established her Harper Method salon franchise in 1891—or the Hall's Hair Renewer (plate 27), or the Seven Sutherland Sisters. These latter actually began their careers in the 1880s, traveling as singers with Barnum and Bailey's Greatest Show on Earth. But their real appeal was their amazingly long hair: collectively, the length of their hair measured thirty-seven feet; Victoria's alone weighed about eleven pounds. In 1885, their father began bottling and distributing a tonic called The Seven Sutherland Sisters Hair Grower, with images of the sisters on the labels and in advertising copy. Between 1886 and 1887—using slogans like "Remember! It's the Hair – not the Hat, that makes a Woman Attractive"—they sold $180,000 worth of the new product, and quickly added a scalp cleanser, a comb, and "hair colorators" to their list of successful products. When their business career ended in 1924, as the popularity of the "bob" grew, sales had reached almost $3 million.[17]

By the later nineteenth century, blonde hair was once again in ascendancy, as witnessed by the Pre-Raphaelites' paintings and verse, fairytale heroines, and also by published complaints: an 1867 article in *Leisure Hour* protested the new fashion for lightening hair.[18] But rather than representing the innocent ideal, now often the blonde suggested danger and sexuality. As Henry Wadsworth Longfellow (1807–1882) warned, "Often treachery lies/ Underneath the fairest hair."[19] But the sense of blonde innocence also prevailed, as in Christina Rossetti's 1862 poem *Goblin Market*, illustrated by her brother Dante, where blonde Laura, enticed by the evil goblins to buy their fruits nightly, pays by cutting and giving them her golden hair. As she sinks deeper and deeper into temptation and sin, her glorious hair grayed and "dwindled," until finally her sister Lizzie rescues her.

Besides the return to blondeness, other major changes occurred with regard to women's hair at the end of the nineteenth century. Up until this time, women had cared for their hair in their own residences, assisted by male *coiffeurs* or female house servants, if wealthy, or by family if not. Now in the later 1800s the first women's public salons began to open, arising literally millennia after men had been regularly using barbershops for everything from their personal grooming and surgical needs to political mongering. Because long wavy hair was preferred, Marcel Grateau in the 1880s in Paris introduced the "Marcel wave," a system using curlers and heated irons without chemicals, and Karl Nessler followed in 1906 in London with the first permanent wave machine; Nessler later established himself at a salon in New York under the name Charles Nestlé. His device, which used electrified rods and curlers dangling down on wires, was both expensive and dangerous; probably it was not much different from the machine displayed in this exhibition. Drying such long hair was of course an issue, and innovative hair dryers proliferated, some using boiling water contained in a metal brush-like tool that heated the hair and claimed to dry it in minutes rather than hours, and others relying on newly available electricity.

Perhaps the most notable revolution in women's hair occurred in the early twentieth century, with the introduction of the bob.[20] Rarely had women worn short hair in western culture. It is reported that Antoine of Paris, in 1910, styled the first bob for actress Eve Lavallière, making her appear immediately younger; by 1913 the famous ballroom dancer Irene Castle was the first well-known American with a bob, followed by the sensational Josephine Baker and others in the 1920s.[21] With regard to bobbed hair, the word "revolution" is no hyperbole: the church, the business world, and even husbands objected to the bob: stories read, "Bobbed hair leads to suit for divorce," and "Shocked husband shoots himself when wife bobs her hair."[22] Women, responding to the liberating freedom brought by short, easy-to-care-for hair, replied: "Unlike Samson who lost his strength in losing his mane, we may gain total power in cutting our hair"[23]: what was emasculation for men became emancipation for women. In the post-war decades, women of all classes turned to the bob, whether because they were busy working women who welcomed its ease, they appreciated it as representing political and social liberation, or they simply liked the style. At about the same time women threw off their corsets, shortened their dresses, and adopted more casual and boyish styles by designers like Coco Chanel of Paris. A whole new definition of "the modern woman" pervaded European and American society, as seen in Edward McCartan's *Portrait of a Young Woman* (plate 29) in terra cotta or Wheeler Williams's bronze *Portrait of Sylvia* from 1923 (plate 28). The fresh boyishness of the former and hints of clean modern abstraction in the latter became the hallmarks of this new American creature who not only voted, but would gain additional social freedoms as the century progressed.

However, this new woman dangerously blurred gender distinctions, both physically and socially, as suggested by this 1927 male complaint: "The species feels itself endangered by a growing inversion. No more hips, no more breasts, no more hair."[24] Others predicted baldness would follow the bobbing, along with the end of motherhood and inability to nurse babies, and generally associated the style with infertility. A Catholic pamphlet warned, "Your children will suffer because of you, and the future generation, product of an age of pleasure, will not know to conserve what our soldiers have defended."[25] Clearly, the human race was about to end, with hair once more at the center of a debate regarding womanhood, manhood, and social and political liberation. For many women, however, the bob became "the clearest symbol of female emancipation."[26]

In 1920, F. Scott Fitzgerald published in the *Saturday Evening Post* his short story "Bernice Bobs Her Hair," a satiric tale of a hopelessly inept eighteen-year-old from Wisconsin who, caving in to peer pressure, gets a liberating but not fully successful "remake" from her selfish cousin out East. Soon after, America's sweetheart, Mary Pickford, joined the bandwagon of the newly emancipated. Long celebrated in movies as virginal "Sweet Little Mary Pickford" and shown with long, brunette ringlets curling down over her bodice, in the 1920s she shifted her image to a more updated, modern woman by not only bleaching her tresses blonde, but styling her hair into the fashionable short bob. Despite the risk of so dramatically altering her public image, she won a best actress Oscar for her aptly-named first talkie, *Coquette*, where she played a flirtatious southern socialite in a blonde bob.

In 1925 Anita Loos wrote *Gentlemen Prefer Blondes*. Not only was her heroine Lorelei Lee boyishly bobbed—as illustrated in the first edition by Ralph Barton—demonstrating her liberation from social conventions, but her blondeness functioned as a synthesis of the innocent, pure, youthful but sexy stereotypes of preceding centuries. Amusingly, the famous Lorelei from German literature was a siren with long golden tresses whose music seduced sailors and led them to their deaths in the Rhine; this Lorelei, with her bobbed blonde good looks and gold-digger mentality, was perhaps even more dangerous, especially to wealthy men.

Hollywood quickly picked up on the blonde craze. The appearance of "the blonde bombshell" Jean Harlow in the movie *Platinum Blonde* in 1931 encouraged American women to try the double-process blonding system developed in the 1920s that led to the clearly artificial color, platinum blonde. No longer was there any subtlety about being blonde, nor pretense of naturalness; now the color was clearly chemically created. Harlow, who died at age twenty-six, so abused her hair with peroxide, household bleach, soap flakes, and ammonia, that she eventually had to resort to a wig.[27] Other platinum screen stars mixed comedy with a blend of innocence and sex, and over time the "fast-talking dames" or "dizzy blondes" of the 1930s, such as Mae West, Carole Lombard, and Ginger Rogers, were replaced by the "dumb blondes" of post-war America: Judy Holliday, Carol Channing, and Marilyn Monroe.[28] The latter two both revived the role of Lorelei Lee, Channing on Broadway in 1949, and Monroe in the 1953 movie co-starring Jane Russell.

For many, of course, Marilyn Monroe remains the quintessential blonde of the twentieth century. Born a brunette, Monroe dyed her hair "Dirty Pillow Slip" blonde, and became the sensation of 1950s Hollywood. Relying on the same colorist who produced Jean Harlow's sensational peroxide tresses, Monroe best embodied the dumb blonde, one symptom of the post-war backlash against increasingly independent women.[29] Acutely aware of her physical features, Monroe realized her face was covered with unusually downy, silvery hair, quite visible in Philippe Halsman's 1952 photograph. She took pains to manipulate lighting, makeup, and accessories to enhance its luminous effect on her skin.[30]

Hair coloring companies played a major role in the transformation of women to blondes, with L'Oréal (founded by Eugene Schueller in 1911) dominating the European market, and Clairol (founded by Lawrence Gelb in 1931) the American. In 1950 Clairol developed a combination bleaching and coloring one-step process for those wishing to lighten their hair only several shades—peroxide was still necessary for major color shifts. Their 1950s ad campaign, with the famous slogan "Does she or doesn't she? Hair color so natural only her hairdresser knows for sure," created sales in the millions, and encouraged women to take the plunge and test their other teaser: "Is it true blondes have more fun?" Clairol followed this up in the 1960s with the astonishingly successful "If I have but one life to live, let me live it as a blonde."[31] While it is estimated that only between 5 and 17 percent of American women are natural blondes, more than 40 percent of American women process their hair to be blonde. Even in Japan, 25 percent of L'Oreal's hair coloring products now sold are for producing blonde hair. The advent of do-it-yourself products greatly expanded women's and men's desires to color their hair, in an industry that today reaps $1.4 billion a year—with the men's coloring market growing twice as fast as the women's.[32]

Breck took advantage of the blonde craze when creating an advertising campaign for their liquid shampoo, invented in 1908. In 1936, Edward Breck, son of the founder, commissioned artist Charles Sheldon to create oil and pastel portraits of striking women, most of them blonde, including the first Breck Girl Roma Whitney, who became the famous profile in the company's logo. Sheldon continued to produce these idealized images of the perfect American girl until succeeded by Ralph Williams, who finally in 1974, under the influence of the civil rights and Black is Beautiful movements, portrayed the first African-American Breck Girl. In a remarkable advertising shift, Donna Alexander, a veterinary student at the University of Pennsylvania, sports a modest Afro while promoting Gold Formula Breck. As home hair care products proliferated—dyes, perms, gels, conditioners—the whole fashion scene became increasing democratized.

Hair color matters, as research confirms. Blonde females, whether natural or dyed, are represented in higher numbers than they appear in real life in literature, the media, and even Miss America contests, and are clearly associated with positive concepts like beauty, innocence, purity, perfection, and youth.[33] With regard to the last, infants are frequently blonde, and only later develop darker tresses. Thus being blonde realizes western societies' goal of perpetual youthfulness, but also may feed male desires for women who appear controllable. In the Renaissance, women typically married at about age fifteen or sixteen, while men averaged twenty-eight or thirty; men were thus significantly more mature and experienced than their wives and could better function as heads of household. For some, blondeness may reflect those halcyon days of childlike women. By contrast, redheads, perhaps because of their relative rarity and sense of difference, since the time of ancient Greece and Rome have been associated with negative stereotypes, including the wearing of red wigs by Roman actors playing slaves and the tradition for clowns to be red-headed: comedienne Lucille Ball's dyed hair and Bozo's red wig (plate 51) are actually part of a long tradition of seeing red-heads as foolish and predictably out-of-control.[34]

1. M. Madou, "Cornes et Cornettes," *Flanders in a European Perspective*, ed. M. Smeyers and B. Cardon (Louvain: Uitgeverij Peeters, 1995), 417–426.

2. Joanna Woods-Marsden, "Portrait of the Lady, 1430–1520," in *Virtue and Beauty*, ed. David Brown (Washington: National Gallery of Art, 2001), 67.

3. See Joseph Manca, "Blond Hair as a Mark of Nobility in Ferrarese Portraiture of the Quattrocento," *Musei Ferraresi* 17 (1990/1991), 51–60.

4. According to *Glamour* magazine, as quoted in Barnaby Conrad, *The Blonde* (San Francisco: Chronicle Books, 1999), 25.

5. *Rime sparse*, as quoted in Joanna Pitman, *On Blondes* (London: Bloomsbury, 2003), 71; from *Petrarch's Lyric Poems: The* Rime sparse *and Other Lyrics*, trans. and ed. Robert M. Durling (Cambridge, Mass.: Harvard University Press, 1976), 100 and 136.

6. Konrad Eisenbichler and Jacqueline Murray, trans. and eds., *On the Beauty of Women* (Philadelphia: University of Pennsylvania Press, 1992), 45.

7. See Pitman, *On Blondes*, 98–102; and Richard Corson, *Fashions in Hair: The First Five Thousand Years* (London: Peter Owen, 1971), 172–174.

8. *Anatomie of Abuses*, 3rd ed. (1585; reprint, London: W. Pickering, 1836), 60–61.

9. Corson, *Fashions in Hair*, 171.

10. Mary Trasko, *Daring Do's: A History of Extraordinary Hair* (Paris: Flammarion, 1984), 34.

11. Trasko, *Daring Do's*, 67.

12. On these satires, see Diana Donald, *The Age of Caricature* (New Haven and London: Yale University Press, 1996), especially chapter 3.

13. For changes in dress and hair style in revolutionary France, see in particular Paul Gerbod, *Histoire de la Coiffure et des Coiffeurs* (Paris: Larousse, 1995), 132–135 and 155–160; and Valerie Steele, *Paris Fashion: A Cultural History*, 2nd ed. (Oxford and New York: Berg, 1998), 43–53.

14. For information on *Godey's* and other fashion magazines, see *Eighty* Godey's *Full-Color Fashion Plates: 1838–1880*, ed. JoAnne Olian (Mineola, N.Y.: Dover Pubs., 1998), iii–v. *Godey's* was founded in 1830 by Louis Antoine Godey, who brought in Mrs. Sarah Josepha Hale to serve as editor from 1837 to 1877. She, the first female editor in the United States and friend of both Emma Willard and Harriet Beecher Stowe, had already been editing *The Ladie's Magazine*, which Godey bought.

15. See Corson, *Fashions in Hair*, 472–485.

16. Trasko, *Daring Do's*, 97.

17. I thank Brandon Stickney for information on the Sutherlands.

18. Corson, *Fashions in Hair*, 480, quotes from that article.

19. Quoted in Wendy Cooper, *Hair: Sex, Society, Symbolism* (New York: Stein and Day, 1971), 76.

20. On the bob, see Mary Louise Roberts, "Samson and Delilah Revisited: The Politics of Women's Fashion in 1920s France," *The American Historical Review* 98 (1993): 657–684.

21. Trasko, *Daring Do's*, 109. Other writers believe the bob was established only after World War I, when indeed the new style became popular.

22. Trasko, *Daring Do's*, 111.

23. French feminist Henriette Sauret, who also called short hair "a gesture of independence." See Roberts, "Samson and Delilah Revisited," 664 and 662.

24. Roberts, "Samson and Delilah Revisited," 670, quoting literary critic Pierre Lièvre.

25. Roberts, "Samson and Delilah Revisited," 671–672, refering to Dr. François Fouveau de Courmelles in 1919, and quoting a natalist Catholic pamphlet from 1920.

26. Roberts, "Samson and Delilah Revisited," 676, quoting journalist Paul Reboux, 1927.

27. Pitman, *On Blondes*, 207.

28. On these earlier blonde bombshells, see Maria DiBattista, *Fast-Talking Dames* (New Haven and London: Yale University Press, 2001), especially 85–131, and her discussion of "Blondes Born Yesterday," 325–335.

29. Pitman, *On Blondes*, 225–226.

30. I thank David Shayt for pointing this out to me in the Christie's 1999 sales catalogue of Monroe memorabilia.

31. See Conrad, *The Blonde*, 39–43 and 25, on the Clairol ads and development.

32. See Conrad, *The Blonde*, 25–27; Stanley Frank, "Brunette Today, Blonde Tomorrow," *Saturday Evening Post*, 9 September 1961, 20–21 and 45; and Bruce Horovitz, "Sales Spotlight Blond Ambition," in *USA Today*, 27 August 2001.

33. Melissa K. Rich and Thomas F. Cash, "The American Image of Beauty: Media Representations of Hair Color for Four Decades," *Sex Roles* 29 (1993): 113–124.

34. On red hair, see Ruth Mellinkoff, "Judas's Red Hair and the Jews," *Journal of Jewish Art* 9 (1982): 31–46, as well as her chapter on hair in *Outcasts: Signs of Otherness in Northern European Art of the Late Middle Ages* (Berkeley: University of California Press, 1993); and Dennis E. Clayson and Micol R. C. Maughan, "Redheads and Blonds: Stereotypic Images," *Psychological Reports* 59 (1986): 811–816.

HAIR
POWER

Penny Howell Jolly

DANGEROUS HAIR

TRESSES OF WOMEN'S HAIR have long signaled women's power to entrap men, as seen in the literary and visual arts, as well as in popular culture. It is a motif that repeats throughout western culture, not just since the Renaissance.

While biblical accounts make no mention of Eve's hair, artists frequently depict her with sinuous curls, alluding to the popular notion that Eve seduced Adam into sin: a narrative element not present in the original Genesis text. We see such an Eve in Albrecht Dürer's *Fall of Man* from 1504: while the anatomically perfect Eve and Adam stand unmoving in an Eden where no tree leaf even whispers with movement, Eve's long, curly hair capriciously flows out behind her, as though blown by some unseen wind that disturbs nothing else. Sinuous and curving like the serpent, her hair forms an entangling trap for Adam. John Milton's description of Eve reveals her as a blonde, and her hair foreshadows the serpent entwining the Tree of Knowledge: "She, as a veil down to the slender waist/ Her unadorned golden tresses wore/ Disheveled, but in wanton ringlets waved,/ As the vine curls her tendrils, which implied/ Subjection, but required with gentle sway."[1] Shakespeare's Bassanio in *The Merchant of Venice* imagines that Portia's hair could be "A golden mesh t' entrap the hearts of men/ Faster than gnats in cobwebs."[2] The German poet Goethe, in his 1810 *Faust*, has Mephistopheles warn of Lilith: "Beware/ That lovely hair of hers, those tresses/Which she incomparably de-lights to wear!/ The young man whom she lures into their snare/ She will not soon release from her caresses."[3]

The association of sinful women with entangling hair is found as well in images of Mary Magdalene, although her hair transforms in meaning over the course of her saintly narrative. At first, it marks her worldly and sensual nature, since she was popularly understood to have been a prostitute. But hair is also the vehicle of her transformation, for she uses it in her penance and humility to wash Christ's feet. Later, after she has exiled herself to a solitary and possessionless existence in the desert, her hair confirms her sanctity, as it grows miraculously to cover her nakedness. Albrecht Dürer's woodcut of the *Assumption of Mary Magdalene* shows her in this final stage of life, as angels transport her daily in order to feed on celestial fare. But her hair retains this triple significance that encapsulates her story: sin, penitential cleansing, and rebirth.

By contrast, Edvard Munch's *The Sin* from 1902 shows no such transformation. Shameless, a half-length female stands naked before the viewer, her luxuriant red hair tousled and hanging unkempt down to her waist. Red hair has consistently been seen as a negative in western tradition and on females frequently suggests dangerous and untrustworthy sexuality and lust; it was even believed a mark of witches. Her disheveled state reaffirms her uncontrolled nature. Even in Ireland, where a large percentage of the world's population of redheads lives, popular folklore warns, "To meet a red-haired woman is a sure omen of misfortune."[4] And despite the ascent of stars like Rita Hayworth, an "exotic" Latina whose sexuality and stardom were enhanced when she dyed her hair red—as for her famous 1946 "Put the Blame on Mame" number—research shows that today redheads still carry negative stereotypes.[5]

Associating the femme fatale with long, unbound hair remains a commonplace in the western tradition, and among its longest-lived examples are versions of the Medusa myth.[6] Even Vik Muniz's light-hearted photographic reworking in pasta and marinara sauce of Caravaggio's painting of the ancient myth—his *Medusa Marinara* from 1999—evokes the horror associated with viewing directly the dangerous and literally "fatale" Medusa. Anyone who beheld her serpent hair turned to stone. Other examples of women who were fatally attractive—the Sirens, the Rhinegold Maidens—similarly had entangling hair that led men to their deaths, as seen in Aubrey Beardsley's illustrations for Wagner's *Das Rheingold* in the December 1896 edition of the *Savoy*. At about the same time, Beardsley also illustrated Oscar Wilde's *Salome*, where the highly sexed Salome has just performed her dance of the seven veils in order to seduce Herod into beheading John the Baptist. In his famous image, Salome's serpentine hair reaches upward like tentacles, at the same time seemingly dripping to the floor, like the blood that flows from John's severed neck. The play between serpents, hair, and blood at the moment that Salome kisses the Baptist's head mixes sexuality and bloodthirstiness in a terrible tangle of danger and carnality.

The association of removal of hair with the stripping of power is another consistent theme, for both women and men. It can be depicted in a humorous light, as in Hogarth's *A Midnight Modern Conversation* (plate 21). The drunken reveler at the rear, toasting with his glass, has removed his wig, visible in his left hand. Given the connotations of masculine authority and class associated with wigs, their inappropriate removal was a certain sign of impotency. But far more humiliating is the practice, found throughout history, of forced removal of hair as a punishment or as a signal of defeat, for example, when vanquished foes are shaved by conquerors. While sometimes other reasons may be proffered—improved hygiene in prisons, or ease of equipment wearing in the military—nonetheless, when a prisoner's or new recruit's hair is shaved almost to the scalp, the message of authority and power is clear: we control you. Following World War II, suspected collaborators on both sides were punished and shamed by public shaving, especially women who were believed to have consorted with the enemy, whether Allied or Axis. A broadside in Linz warned: "We'll watch you on the street, we'll cut your hair, and we'll tear off your clothes and send you running naked for home."[7] Robert Capa's famous photograph of a Nazi collaborator captures the venomous hostility of this aggressive action, which typically involved more than just cutting by scissors. By contrast, as a consensual act, for example following religious practices, the self-inflicted shaving of hair can indicate celibacy or self-denial, thus a voluntary sacrifice to a higher power.

But certainly the most famous narrative of power-wielding hair and its forcible removal is that of Samson from the Book of Judges in the Old Testament. At first, Samson's hairiness signals his extreme virility and unnatural strength: body and head hair grew prolifically, it was believed, due to heat produced in men; colder and moister women suffered a deficiency in this area, and thus were relatively hairless and hence weak. Such ancient beliefs may figure in modern men's fear of baldness. Thus in Dürer's *Samson Fighting the Lion* woodcut, the hero's hirsute appearance assures the viewer of his eventual victory: the lion, while overall more hairy, remains a beast, and Samson's physical and moral superiority remains clear. Yet, while more than a match for the lion, Samson is defeated—as the story is popularly told, although not as recounted in Judges 16—by the wiles of a woman who seduces him and cuts off his hair, leaving him symbolically castrated. Interestingly, in Gustave Doré's illustrated bible from 1874, when Delilah approaches Samson he already appears "castrated," in that Doré has feminized him: Samson leans languidly on a seat while pulling on his luxuriant tresses, exposing a prominent earring; by contrast, Delilah stands, her head and body modestly veiled.

BODY HAIR

The prepubescent child eagerly awaits the arrival of body hair: girls typically grow pubic hair around age eleven, and axillary hair soon follows; boys of about twelve begin sprouting pubic hair, followed in the next three or four years by chest and body hair, and finally within another year by facial hair. As a biological marker of maturity, development of body hair is almost unparalleled. What we then do with it culturally—how we manipulate it by growing it here and shaving or waxing it there—reflects many of our socially and politically formed ideas about who we are. The degree to which images reflect real social practices is difficult to determine, however, as artists' handling of body hair is conditioned by artistic conventions and meanings, and may not reflect actual body hair management.

The practice of shaving body hair is largely a twentieth-century development, although early western cultures from the Egyptian to the Roman practiced it. Ancient Egyptians valued smooth, hairless bodies for both women and men, and utilized abrasives like pumice to effect that result. Pubic depilation—whether by singeing or plucking—was practiced in ancient Greece, although vase paintings of prostitutes, or even sexualized scenes of rape, were likely to include pubic hair as an erotic element.[8] But for the Christian Middle Ages, evidence of body hair removal seems absent, although some suggest that aristocratic women for a time beginning in the late Middle Ages practiced pubic depilation, influenced by Crusaders returning from Muslim harems. In the Renaissance, there is some evidence for this practice. Jean de la Montagne in 1525 remarked that to be elegant, a woman should be completely shaven, while Erasmus, writing his 1509 *In Praise of Folly*, mocks old women who "pluck and thin their pubic bush."[9] However, pubic depilation was apparently ended by Catherine de'Medici, Queen of France, in the mid-sixteenth century.[10] No evidence suggests removal of hair from underarms or legs.

In the Renaissance, artists like Dürer and Hans Baldung Grien depicted witches, as the anti-witchcraft craze hit Europe by the early sixteenth century, and prominent hair is one of their signs. Baldung's *Witches' Sabbath* of 1510 shows six naked witches brewing their infernal potions, surrounded by pitchforks, bones, and their familiars: two goats and a cat. Whether they are flying through the air or stirring their pots, their long hair whips out behind them, signaling their potent sexuality. It was believed that, in order to fly, witches would rub the staffs of their pitchforks or their own bodies with nefarious potions "under the arms and in other hairy places."[11] According to the 1487 *Malleus maleficarum (The Witches' Hammer)*, a Dominican text explaining how to combat witchcraft, when a suspected witch was arrested, the first act should be to shave her entire body. Clearly the removal of all body and head hair by inquisitors was an attempt to diminish the unnatural creatures' powers. This may be why some sixteenth-century images of witches, including Baldung's famous painting *Weather Witches* in Frankfurt, are among the very rare Renaissance depictions of axillary—that is, underarm—hair, and also frequently show pubic hair.

Even women who were not witches, if they were "rough and thick grown with hair" in their "secret privities," were judged insatiable for sex by nature, even lecherous.[12] We see this association between pubic hair and vain earthly pleasures in later art, for example in Castellan's print of Edgar Allan Poe's *Masque of the Red Death*, where a female figure with luxuriant pubic hair and grotesque head represents one of the wanton phantasms or dreams present at Prince Prospero's "voluptuous" masquerade.

The shaping or total depilation of women's pubic hair, a trend increasingly popular today in this country, could, like the blonde ideal, be a symbolic depowering of women: such denuding does infantilize mature bodies. By contrast, contemporary artist Millie Wilson, in her *Museum of Lesbian Dreams* from 1990–1992, pays particular attention to female pubic hair and empowers it by literally enhancing it. In one section of the work, *Merkins*, she makes a series of elaborately curled and manipulated wigs, each named for a different woman. Merkins, a term probably derived from "maulkin," itself a slang term for a lower class woman, are pubic wigs worn by women—usually prostitutes originally—at least as early as the seventeenth century, possibly to cover signs of disease, to replace hair lost in illness, or to cover bald pudenda shaved in an effort to reduce lice. Today, merkins most typically are worn in theatrical and cinematic circumstances as a modesty cover, by cancer patients to replace hair lost due to radiation therapy, or for erotic enhancement. In another part of her *Museum*, Wilson again focuses on female genitalia, but this time making a visual play between a typology of eighteenth-century male wigs, itself a satire by Hogarth included separately in this exhibition (plate 5), and an actual page from Dr. George W. Henry's 1948 *Sex Variants: A Study of Homosexual Patterns*, his search for deviant physical manifestations of homosexuality in female genitalia. Using a reproduction of a Louis XIV style wig in the center to link the two taxonomies of male wigs and female genitals, she juxtaposes these images of supposed authority and power. Hogarth mocks the "bigwig"; Wilson similarly reveals to the viewer the ridiculousness of Henry's no-longer authoritative typology that claimed deviance. This suggestion of "inversion," a psychiatric term used in the past for homosexuality, subverts the power of both images, and at the same time empowers lesbian sexuality.[13]

The typical Renaissance nude in art generally lacks pubic hair, although exceptions exist, particularly among works by Flemish and German artists and in depictions of males, for example, Michelangelo's *David*.[14] In some images, visual body hair seems simply to result from the meticulously detailed style of an artist: Jan van Eyck's almost life-sized, virtuoso Adam and Eve in the Ghent Altarpiece of 1432 sport not only pubic hair, but also leg and arm hair, wrinkles, fingernails, surface veins, and other body details often omitted by artists. Dürer depicted pubic hair on both Adam and Eve in his engraving, a somewhat unusual choice, as more commonly pubic hair is included in images more openly stressing excessive sexuality than these: besides witches, images of Venus, Vanitas, the goddesses in the Judgment of Paris, or other sensual women—even including Lucretia, who is raped.

However, the academic tradition for depicting males and especially females with fully idealized, hairless bodies continues into the nineteenth and twentieth centuries, even though by then many artists routinely eschewed academic notions of beauty. In this exhibition, we see smooth-bodied, academic nudes in Benjamin West's classically inspired 1803 *Venus Lamenting the Death of Adonis* (plate 42) and in Mario Joseph Korbel's lovely marble *Female Torso* from 1927 (plate 44). In this sculpture, the white of the marble reinforces the ideally smoothed flesh, as no hint of imperfection—or hair!—is created. What a contrast, then, with Edward Kienholz's *Bunny, Bunny, You're So Funny* (plate 45), an assemblage that was censored in 1963 and removed from an exhibition at San Fernando Valley State College.[15] Kienholz aggressively mixes the organic female form with sharp metallic materials, as his nude half torso wears chicken-wire red mesh stockings held up by metal garters, and its amputated limbs end in metal doorknobs instead of feet. The torso itself is supported by a metal stand, and contains a plastic baby doll that can be spun by a mechanical crank appended to the hip of the figure. But perhaps most shocking of all is the figure's pubic hair: it is formed from steel-wool.

Another potentially shocking female torso is Birgit Dieker's *Beasty Girl* from 2001 (plate 43): an extremely naturalistically posed woman standing attentively with hands on her hips, her inset blue eyes seemingly alive, but whose entire body is covered with hair, some human and some sheep's wool.[16] Quite in contrast to Korbel's sensual *Torso*, which is raised on a pedestal even while tempting the viewer to touch it, *Beasty Girl* subverts the traditional idealized female nude by substituting a frighteningly monstrous form: life-sized and in our space. But Dieker also here returns to her Germanic roots, for there a tradition exists, especially popular in late medieval and Renaissance Germany, for depicting Wild Men and Women. We see these for example in Martin Schongauer's engravings from about 1470, which even include a Wild Woman nursing a small Wild Child. The meaning of these hirsute figures varies over time, but in Schongauer's day was generally relatively positive, quite unlike our werewolf horror fantasies.[17] These wild people, although less than human, are natural people, associated with superhuman strength and virility (the males) and fecundity and fertility (the females). Schongauer's tamed examples, both of whom support coats-of-arms, are subservient to their noble "masters" and transfer to them their protection, strength, and promise of fertility.

For many contemporary women, hairless bodies remain the ideal, and shaving or waxing a regular ritual. Except among feminists, some of whom refuse to remove body hair, American women typically shave both their axillary and leg hair; bikini waxes are also increasingly popular. But these are relatively recent developments, widespread only post-World War II, and it is ironic that the "smoothing" of underarms and legs, as it was often called in the 1910s and 1920s, dates to the era when women began bobbing their hair as a sign of liberation.

Newfound freedom in one arena of personal hygiene thus left women open to slavish attention in another. The first push for the shaving of underarms began in May of 1915, when ads in *Harper's Bazaar* alerted women to problems of unsightly hair occasioned by the new, sleeveless fashions; these were soon followed by ads concerning "limbs."[18] When Sears marketed dresses with sheer sleeves for the first time in 1922, they simultaneously offered a woman's décolleté safety razor, a slightly smaller version of a man's, in different packaging.[19] Advertising encouraging hairless legs continued into the 1920s, "necessitated" by short skirts, sheer stockings, and more revealing bathing costumes; but, as with the boyish bob from the '20s, moral issues concerning "bad" women discouraged some. Nevertheless, by World War II sexy legs were in, and they needed to be hairless; by 1964, 98 percent of American women aged fifteen to forty-four removed body hair.[20] Not until the women's movements of the late 1960s and 1970s did women refuse to shave for ideological reasons. Indeed, shaving of body hair not only heightens sexual difference, but simultaneously infantilizes women, making their bodies once again seem eternally youthful and immature.[21] At exactly the periods when women were becoming freer—the 1920s with its unisex styling, the 1940s with Rosie the Riveter—pressure was increased to keep women feminine.

THREADING HAIRS OF MEMORY AND MOURNING

It should not be surprising that hair fulfills many roles relevant to memorializing deceased persons, given its malleability on the living and durability following death. Many cultures worldwide prescribe hair rituals when mourning the dead, such as purposeful deranging of the hair by pulling, cutting, or even shaving. Hair itself is already dead as soon as it has grown from the follicle, so even when cut from the body of the deceased, it retains its color and form over centuries. As a writer in the 1850 volume of *Godey's Lady's Book* noted, "Hair is at once the most delicate and lasting of our materials and survives us like love."

Hair is also intimate and personal: we don't share our hair with our friends, nor touch other people's hair, except in especially close relationships. Thus cutting a lock from one's lover is akin to acknowledging intimacy. When Robert Browning asked Elizabeth Barrett for "what I have always dared to think I would ask you for...a lock of your hair," she replied, "I never gave away what you ask me to give you, to a human being, except my nearest relatives & once or twice or thrice to female friends."[22] He did eventually receive that treasure. Locks of both Brownings are included in this exhibition (plates 36 and 37), from a *Collection of Hair* compiled by English poet and friend of John Keats, J. H. Leigh Hunt (1784–1859).

Alexander Pope's famous mock-epic poem *The Rape of the Lock* depends upon implied sexual violence incurred by the unauthorized taking of a lock of hair. Pope's satire derives from an incident in 1711, when Robert, Lord Petre, clipped hair from an unmarried twenty-two-year-old, Arabella Fermor (fictionalized as the Baron and Belinda, respectively, in the poem). First written in 1712 at the request of John Caryll, a relative of Lord Petre, and dedicated to Ms. Fermor, the poem was conceived as a means of lending humor to a tense situation and relieving stress between the two families. Pope revised and expanded his comic-heroic epic in 1714 and again in 1717 and published—under a pseudonym—the *Key to the Lock*, a mock critique of his own work. In Aubrey Beardsley's illustration for the April 1896 *Savoy*, the Baron steals up behind the innocent Belinda, and reaches toward her elaborately curled hair. It is, of course, the intimacy associated with hair—"th' inestimable Prize" becomes the virtue of the young, innocent woman—that makes so intolerable the Baron's act of displaying it in his finger ring to "gazing Eyes."[23] Indeed, it was already customary in mid-seventeenth-century England for lovers to exchange rings with locks of hair.

Many pieces of jewelry embellished with human hair functioned as mourning jewelry (plates 38–41), examples of which are included in this exhibition. In the seventeenth century, people wore *memento-mori* rings encasing hair and inscribed with the date and name or initials of the deceased, while in the later eighteenth and early nineteenth centuries, women wore mourning brooches and pendants as well.[24] Hair in these could take the form of locks formed into a curl; plaited, woven, or twisted strands of hair; or even hair that was dissolved or ground up, mixed with the paint medium, and used for painting allegorical scenes with willow trees, tombstones, and other motifs symbolic of mourning. Such jewelry became astonishingly popular in the nineteenth century, especially during the Civil War in this country and in England following the 1861 death of Queen Victoria's beloved Prince Albert. Victoria gave and received countless gifts of hair tokens, many memorializing Albert, but others using her own hair. As one popular rhyme expressed, "If I should from this world/ Depart you'd have a bit of my/ Hair my hand and heart if we/ Could no more each other see/ You could still remember me."[25] Perhaps the most ambitious example of hairwork associated with Victoria was a life-sized portrait of the queen, entirely of hair, exhibited at the Paris Exposition of 1855.[26]

By the second half of the nineteenth century, changes in fashion and technique produced hair jewelry that allowed the hair to touch the body of the wearer directly. Following cleansing of the hair by boiling it in borax and water and then scraping it, hair workers wove a few strands of hair at a time, weighted on a weaving table, over variously designed molds made of wood, wire, or metal. Formed into openwork patterns, the hair dried into hollow geometrical shapes that could be glued and attached to gold fittings, then made into earrings, bracelets, necklaces, or watch chains. While one could provide friends' or relatives' hair, manufactured pieces were often created from hair purchased from convents or lower class women selling their hair to earn money; the makers were professional jewelers, some of whom became quite famous for this specialty. But women also learned to make hair jewelry. For example, the popular *Godey's Lady's Book* from December 1850 included the first published instructions in America for making hairwork on a home braiding table, and one of the device's selling points was that the owner could be assured of the hair's authenticity.[27]

Making one's own hair wreath similarly assured the accurate identification of the hair, as women's skills included forming delicate flowers from their own family's tresses and mounting them onto shaped bases. Hair was collected daily from combs and brushes and placed in personal receptacles called hair receivers; several examples are in this exhibition. Popular particularly in later nineteenth-century America, these large hair wreaths were constructed over a period of time, eventually memorializing generations within a family. Framed in boxes and displayed in domestic settings, some were even provided with labels or diagrams identifying each flower's source. Although generally made while the donors were living, over time these hair wreaths became memorials to the deceased. But by the early twentieth century the practice faded, partly due to fears of contagion, as the hair began to be considered unhealthy; many examples of hairwork were burned.

Hair of famous individuals has long fascinated historical and literary buffs. An interesting example of the nineteenth-century obsession with hair is the album compiled by J. H. Leigh Hunt, parts of which are on display (plates 35–37). Hunt, part of the Romantic circle of writers, focuses in particular upon the literary giants of his day— Keats, the Shelleys, Wordsworth, Charles Lamb—but also includes other famous figures: Napoleon and George Washington.

It is interesting here to juxtapose the iconic portrait of the first American president, one of Gilbert Stuart's own replicas of his original from 1795–1796 (plate 34), with a lock of George Washington's actual hair. Which is the more potent visual experience? Which creates a more powerful sense of presence? Washington himself refused to wear a wig, associating it with upper class ambitions, and was dismayed that Martha, a wealthy woman when he married her, was ordering wigs from France. We see him in Stuart's portrait wearing his own hair, now white and perhaps powdered, styled in a simple *queue*, similar to wigs of the period; replicas of gentlemen's more elaborate *queue* wigs are included in the exhibition. Hunt's lock of Washington's hair, though, is surprisingly powerful. Like a bone or other bodily fragment displayed for meditation by the faithful in a medieval reliquary, this rare physical remnant of the legendary Father of our Country is met with quiet respect from today's viewers.

Hair is associated with mourning and death in other ways, as it is often manipulated exceptionally at important moments of transition. For example, a male might disregard shaving, thus indicating the suspension of social order during a period of mourning. Similarly, the practice of pulling at, shaving, or even tearing out one's hair as a mourning gesture is an ancient one, especially associated with women.[28] Signaling a clear discontinuance of normal deportment while grieving for a deceased spouse, a married woman in mourning might let her hair down; the bonds of marriage are literally being loosed and disarranged. We see this long-standing western tradition visualized in Benjamin West's marvelous painting *Venus Lamenting the Death of Adonis* from 1803 (plate 42). This goddess of love is no blonde; West had just been to Paris, where dark-haired beauties reigned. She here finds her young lover, Adonis, who has ignored her warnings and been slain by a wild boar; from his blood the anemone sprouts. Overcome with grief, Venus falls to her knees and arches her back; her long sinuous hair, conventionally an expression of her beauty and sexuality, she here pulls out in despair, while her attendants gently restrain her. As Ovid describes, in George Sandys' elegant 1632 edition: "Downe jumping from the skies, at once she tore/ Her haire and bosome: then her brest invades/ With bitter blowe."[29]

HAIRITAGE: AFRICAN-AMERICAN EXPERIENCES.[30]

Hair has always been important to African-Americans, as demonstrated by the ubiquity of hair narratives by contemporary black writers, but also by accounts written about African-American slaves and their particular interest in hair grooming as early as the later eighteenth century.[31] Even before the Civil War, the use of blacksmithing tools as straighteners anticipated the later development of the hot comb (plate 49). Thus long before Madam C. J. Walker's heyday at the opening of the twentieth century, there was a powerful black beauty culture in this country, whether it involved weaving cotton through the prongs of a fork to comb and clean the hair, rubbing chopped corn into the scalp as a cleanser, using lard or butter as a conditioner, or shaving parts of the crown while leaving other hair long and combed up high over the forehead.[32]

Many African-Americans today recount childhood memories of hair toiletry rituals: mothers heating hot combs on a stove, the use of concoctions of grease, the difficulty of dealing with the "kitchen"—the densest hair at the nape of the neck—and the smell of singed hair and tenderness of burned scalps that inevitably occurred.[33] Painful and difficult as these processes sound, for many they formed a rite of passage that cemented their sense of belonging within a community, even as it simultaneously could reflect a desire to appear more like women and men in the mainstream white culture. In 1992, it was estimated that African-Americans purchased 19 percent of all toiletries and cosmetics sold but 34 percent of all hair care products—three times that of other Americans.[34] Even today, an estimated 70–75 percent of black women in the United States straighten their hair.[35]

Beauty products and processes proliferated in the twentieth-century African-American community, and entrepreneurs arose to manufacture those products. Certainly the most famous is Madam C. J. Walker (1867–1919), née Sarah Breedlove, a self-made millionaire who established herself in Indianapolis in 1910, but whose black hair-care and cosmetics products were sold nationally through her franchise: the Madam C. J. Walker Hair Culturists Union of America.[36] She employed thousands of African-Americans as profitable "hair culturists" and sales agents, and became a leader within the black community. Already in the early twentieth century there were voices who spoke against hair straightening, seeing it as reflecting a desire to appear white, and these complaints resurfaced in the black nationalist movements of the 1960s and 1970s. But Madam C. J. Walker, while credited with popularizing the straightening comb around 1905, never used the word "straightener" in her advertisements, instead emphasizing that her products were to encourage hair growth, and also self-esteem: "Right here let me correct the erroneous impression held by some that I claim to straighten hair. I deplore such impressions because I have always held myself out as a hair culturist. I grow hair…I want the great masses of my people to take a greater pride in their appearance."[37]

Photographs of African-Americans from the twentieth century here document the variety of hair styles used by fashionable women and men, most of it straightened or "conked" to create more wavy styles. George Grosz's watercolor of a well-dressed lady on the subway in 1933 shows her wearing the newly fashionable bob from the 1920s, her hair sleek and close to her head; she most likely has straightened her hair. Conking, a process widely used during the big band and jazz eras of the 1930s, '40s, and '50s, derived its name from "conglolene," a mixture of sodium hydroxide (lye) and starch, and was popular for men's hair styling.[38] Kobena Mercer argues the conk was a specifically black hair style, and not one imitative of Caucasian styles.[39]

That hair styling has political overtones for African-Americans is perfectly clear.[40] The Afro, the Bush, the Black Pride movement, Black is Beautiful—all of these reflect the importance of hair and identity, and these concerns continue today, as seen in objects in this exhibition. Nat Mathis (b. 1946), an Afro specialist known as the Bush Doctor, opened his first beauty salon in Washington, D.C., in 1969, and in 1970 patented his special hair-styling aprons, one of which is in this exhibition; he was the first African-American to win the coveted International Hair Styling Competition, in Cairo, in 1981.[41] The Afro, a style long worn by African-Americans, was transformed into a political statement by activists like Angela Davis and the Black Panthers. As A.B. Spelman observed, "Big bushy Afros on the sisters and hardbop in the air…. Hair was pride you could grow."[42] For Gloria Wade-Gayles, "[a]n activist with straight hair was a contradiction. A lie. A joke, really…. I decided to wear an Afro."[43] Lee Hirsche's *Blue Necklace* (plate 46), a portrait of an African-American with the classic Afro, dates from 1973, only one year after Angela Davis was acquitted on charges of murder, kidnapping, and conspiracy. Likely for Hirsche's young sitter, the cut was meaningful. But like earlier political styles, Afros became stylish, and were worn by white Americans as well as black.

Contemporary African-American artists still see hair as a site for cultural discourse and establishment of identity, as seen in many contemporary works. Kerry James Marshall's monumental painting *De Style* (plate 50), from 1993, pictures both well-dressed and casually attired African-American men in a barber shop, surrounded by hair products, mass media images, and their own reflections in the shop's mirror. They look at us looking at them, their strikingly unusual hair styles signaling their individuality and expressing their desire to have "style." Similarly Debra Priestly's *Lookin Glass #4* (plate 52) from 1999 shows consciousness of being looked at, but complicates the question by juxtaposing jars and bottles, such as would hold tonics, with dreadlocks, a "natural" style of hair.

Head and body hair remains one of humans' most important means of expression, whether with regard to issues of identity and class status, politics and gender, or moral character and self-esteem. Believing that what is on the outside reflects what is inside, we manipulate our hair to reveal to others who we are, or at least who we want to be.

1. *Paradise Lost*, 4. 304–308.

2. *Merchant of Venice*, 3.2.122–123, as noted in Elisabeth G. Gitter, "The Power of Women's Hair in the Victorian Imagination," *PMLA* 99 (1984): 936.

3. *Walpurgis Night*, 4119–4123, trans. G. M. Priest (New York: Knopf, 1941), 119. See Virginia M. Allen, "'One Strangling Golden Hair': Dante Gabriel Rossetti's *Lady Lilith*," *Art Bulletin* 66 (1984): 286, on the original text.

4. Ruth Mellinkoff, "Judas's Red Hair and the Jews," *Journal of Jewish Art* 9 (1982): 33 n. 23.

5. See Dennis E. Clayson and Micol R. C. Maughan, "Redheads and Blonds: Stereotypic Images," *Psychological Reports* 59 (1986): 811–816; and Melissa K. Rich and Thomas F. Cash, "The American Image of Beauty: Media Representations of Hair Color for Four Decades," *Sex Roles* 29 (1993): 111–124.

6. See Susan Koslow, "'How Looked the Gorgon Then…': The Science and Poetics of the *Head of Medusa* by Rubens and Snyders," in *Shop Talk: Studies in Honor of Seymour Slive* (Cambridge, Mass.: Harvard University Art Museums, 1995), especially 148, on the connections between serpents and women's hair, including pubic hair.

7. See P. Biddiscombe, "Dangerous Liaisons: The Anti-fraternization Movement in the U.S. Occupation Zones of Germany and Austria, 1945–1948," *Journal of Social History* 34 (2001): 611–647, and 620 for the Linz placard.

8. M. Kilmer, "Genital Phobia and Depilation," *Journal of Hellenic Studies* 102 (1982): 104–112.

9. Trans. Clarence H. Miller (New Haven and London: Yale University Press, 1979), 49.

10. See Wendy Cooper, *Hair: Sex, Society, Symbolism* (New York: Stein and Day, 1971), 114–115. In Islam, according to the *Sunnah* of the Prophet, adult women and men are expected to have clean-shaven underarms and pubic regions.

11. Dale Hoak, "Art, Culture, and Mentality in Renaissance Society: The Meaning of Hans Baldung Grien's *Bewitched Groom* (1544)," *Renaissance Quarterly* 38 (1985): 449, quote from Dominican theologian Jordanes de Bergamo, ca. 1470–71.

12. Levinius Lemnius, *Touchstone of Complexions*, published in London in 1633, as quoted in Anthony Fletcher, *Gender, Sex and Subordination in England 1500–1800* (New Haven: Yale University Press, 1995), 45.

13. I thank Katie Hauser for her suggestions regarding the meaning of this work.

14. Anne Hollander, *Seeing through Clothes* (Berkeley: University of California Press, 1978), 136–148, offers an excellent discussion of conventions regarding the female nude and pubic hair in art.

15. See Gerald Silk, "Censorship and Controversy in the Career of Edward Kienholz," in *Suspended License*, ed. E. Childs (Seattle and London: University of Washington Press, 1998), 259–298.

16. See Ellen Heider, "Autopsy of the Beautiful," in *Birgit Dieker: Kardio* (Berlin: Galerie Volker Diehl, 2002), 12–39.

17. On the complexities of these hirsute beings, see Roger Bartra, *Wild Men in the Looking Glass* (Ann Arbor: University of Michigan Press, 1994).

18. Christine Hope, "Caucasian Female Body Hair and American Culture," *Journal of American Culture* 5 (1982): 93–99, discusses these ads and the history of shaving.

19. Hope, "Caucasian Female Body Hair," 95.

20. Hope, "Caucasian Female Body Hair," 97.

21. Hope, in "Caucasian Female Body Hair," 98–99, discusses gender implications of body hair removal. On women's and men's attitudes toward body hair, see J. M. Lewis, "Caucasian Body Hair Management: A Key to Gender and Species Identification in U. S. Culture?," *Journal of American Culture* 10 (1987): 7–14; and Susan A. Basow, "The Hairless Ideal: Women and Their Body Hair," *Psychology of Women Quarterly* 15 (1991): 83–96, and Basow and Amie C. Braman, "Women and Body Hair: Social Perceptions and Attitudes," *Psychology of Women Quarterly* 22 (1998): 637–645.

22. As quoted in Gitter, "The Power of Women's Hair," 943.

23. Canto IV, 113, 114.

24. Diana Scarisbrick, "A Becoming Mourning," *Country Life* 184 (1990): 58–60, discusses English seventeenth-century rings; Davida T. Deutsch, "Jewelry for Mourning, Love, and France, 1770–1830," *Magazine Antiques* 155 (1999): 566–575, discusses later jewelry and includes additional bibliography.

25. Quoted in Irene G. Navarro, "Hairwork of the Nineteenth Century," *Magazine Antiques* 159 (2001): 485.

26. Gitter, "The Power of Women's Hair," 942.

27. Navarro, "Hairwork of the Nineteenth Century," 492.

28. R. Bartlett, "Symbolic Meanings of Hair in the Middle Ages," *Transactions of the Royal Historical Society* ser. 6, vol. 4 (1994): 53–56, discusses various classical and medieval practices and offers additional sources.

29. *Ovid's Metamorphosis*, ed. K. Hulley and S. Vandersall (Lincoln: University of Nebraska Press, 1970), 473.

30. *Hairitage* was the title of a 2002 exhibition on hair in African-American experience produced by the Amistad Foundation, based at the Wadsworth Atheneum, and co-curated by Deirdre Bibby and William Frank Mitchell.

31. See Shane White and Graham White, "Slave Hair and African American Culture in the Eighteenth and Nineteenth Centuries," *Journal of Southern History* 61 (1995): 45–76, as well as numerous recently published accounts in, among others, *Tenderheaded*, ed. Juliette Harris and Pamela Johnson (New York: Simon and Schuster, 2001); Lisa Jones, *Bulletproof Diva: Tales of Race, Sex, and Hair* (New York: Doubleday, 1994); and Henry Louis Gates's essay "In the Kitchen" from his memoir *Colored People* (New York: Knopf, 1994), 40–49.

32. See Willie Morrow, "A Short History of Early Hair Straightening," in *Tenderheaded*, 125–128, and descriptions of hair on slaves in White and White, "Slave Hair and African American Culture," especially 54–56.

33. See for example Natasha Trethewey, "Hot Comb," or bell hooks, "Straightening Our Hair," both in *Tenderheaded*, 108–109 and 111–116; and Malcolm X's chapter on hair in his *Autobiography of Malcolm X*, with Alex Haley (New York: Ballantine Books, 1965), where he talks about the conking process for making kinky hair wavy.

34. Noliwe M. Rooks, *Hair Raising: Beauty, Culture, and African American Women* (New Brunswick, N.J.: Rutgers University Press, 1996), 117. See also Deborah R. Grayson, "Is it Fake? Black Women's Hair as Spectacle and Spec(tac)ular," *Camera Obscura*, 36 (1995): 13–30.

35. *Tenderheaded*, 95 and 103.

36. Much is published about Walker, including a recent biography by her great-great-granddaughter, A'Lelia Bundles, *On Her Own Ground: The Life and Times of Madam C. J. Walker* (New York, London: Scribner, 2001). See also Rooks, *Hair Raising*, especially 51–74.

37. Quoted in Bundles, *On Her Own Ground*, 268–269.

38. *Tenderheaded*, 102.

39. Kobena Mercer, "Black Hair/Style Politics," in *Out There: Marginalization and Contemporary Cultures*, Russell Ferguson, ed. (Cambridge, Mass.: MIT Press, 1990), 258–261.

40. In addition to Mercer, "Black Hair/Style Politics," 247–264, and other books noted above, see Angela Y. Davis, "Afro Images: Politics, Fashion, and Nostalgia," in

Picturing Us: African American Identity in Photography, ed.
Deborah Willis (New York: The New Press, 1994), 170–179;
and Ayana D. Byrd and Lori L. Tharps, *Hair Story:
Untangling the Roots of Black Hair in America* (New York:
St. Martin's Press, 2001).

41. The Nathaniel Mathis Collection of Barbering and
Beauty Culture is housed in the Smithsonian Institution
Archives.
42. Quoted in *Tenderheaded*, 199.
43. Quoted in Rooks, *Hair Raising*, 6–7.

(H)AIR JORDAN: EXCAVATING HIS ROYAL BALDNESS

Jeffrey O. Segrave

HAIR, AS KOBENA MERCER POIGNANTLY REMINDS US, is "never a straightforward 'fact'" because it is almost always "'worked upon' by human hands."[1] Cut, colored, groomed, and concealed, hair is a social practice that operates within a powerful metaphysical and existential matrix; hairstyles become radical and declarative statements about who we are and about who we conceive ourselves to be as human and social beings. As a result, hair assumes profound symbolic importance, and quotidian discourses about hair constitute complex narratives of identity politics. Recognizing, as Ingrid Banks puts it, that "hair matters,"[2] I want to interrogate one of the quintessential—and certainly most well publicized and photographed—expressions of contemporary hairstyling: namely, Michael Jordan's baldness.

"If Aliens came down to earth, and asked to see the most extraordinary human being in existence," the black political activist Harry Edwards once wrote, "I would show them Michael Jordan. A team of physicists, chemists, and scientists can't explain his athletic performances."[3] Arguably the greatest athlete who ever lived, Jordan has become the embodiment of athletic superstardom. While images of his soaring, windmill dunks, blazing baseline maneuvers, and lane-driving heroics may well define him as what Hoberman calls "the paramount symbol of athleticism in the media age,"[4] his bald head stands as a particularly identifiable feature of his ubiquitous presence. But Jordan's pristine dome is more than a jejune incidental, a mere stylistic irrelevance. Rather, his bald head may be construed as a cultural product that is both constituted by and constitutive of a larger context of relationships characteristic of the American condition at the turn of the twenty-first century. Put another way, Jordan's bald dome is, to use Clifford Geertz's formulation, both a model for reality and a model of reality, a prism through which we can see the contours of several historically defining themes in American history. To interrogate Jordan's bald head is to interrogate African-American style, race relations, and Jordan's role as one of the primary signifiers in the spread of neo-liberal democracy and global capitalism—Michael Jordan as the smiling face on what some have characterized as an insidious western, or even American, cultural imperialism.

In order to uncover what the meanings and submerged political implications are of being or perhaps more poignantly wanting to "be like Mike," I'd like to offer a multidisciplinary analysis of Michael Jordan's bald head, one that acknowledges the rise to pre-eminence of the civilization of the image.[5] Within the postmodern media-scape the consumption of images can and does have real effects. Images, visual texts, and signs continuously flood our perceptual radar screens and shape our everyday experiences, relations, and identities; as Kundera notes: "Imagology is stronger than reality."[6] Moreover, the postmodern culture of the image has subtly but indelibly restructured American politics. Ultimately, then, I want to place my reading of Jordan's baldness within the context of the hypersemiurgic culture of postmodernity and argue that because Michael Jordan's image is associated with—in fact defines—Nike's hyperreal Air Jordan, and because Jordan's bald head is a sort of free-floating signifier that as a defining component of the Jordan brand image has accrued enormous promotional capital, Jordan's baldness has profound implications for both black and white Americans, indeed all Americans.

But let it be noted right from the beginning that MJ is not really bald. He is bald-*ing*, and has been for some time; but he is not bald. Actually, he typically shaves his head twice a week, on Tuesdays and Fridays, with an electric shaver.[7] He is then bald-*ed*. Along with his million-dollar smile, his gold earring, his baggy basketball shorts, and his protruding tongue, Jordan's glistening dome is an integral and indeed defining characteristic of his iconic status. Michael Jordan *with* hair does not seem to be Michael Jordan at all. With hair, Jordan does not seem to be much different than any other super-talented black basketball player.[8] But without hair, he is Air Jordan, the global icon, the ultimate-celebrity athlete, "a one-man corporate conglomerate" as David Halberstam calls him.[9] Without hair, he is Mr. GQ, Michael the beautiful, the quintessential expression of black urban manhood; without hair, he is a "hyperreal commodity sign;"[10] he is in fact an empire of signs,[11] the man who has become a sign of himself, to paraphrase Norman Denzin.[12] Like Lady Diana, Muhammad Ali, or Sir Paul

McCartney, Michael Jordan is famous for being famous, an icon to icons.

Not only does the clean pate look define Michael Jordan as Michael Jordan, it is also one of the defining Afro-American hairstyles of the era, replacing the seemingly inveterate high top fad. Just as Pamela Grier in the blaxploitation movies of the '70s made fashionable a defiant Afro that offered black women a proud, natural appearance, and just as cornrows and braids have been redefined by Philadelphia 76er Allen Iverson, so has Michael Jordan popularized the hairless 'do, transforming it into what might well be the most memorable hair trend of the fin de millennium.[13]

Jordan is certainly not the first great athlete to sport a bald pate. Jack Johnson, the black heavyweight boxing champion of the early twentieth century, shaved his head, as did several of his sparring partners. But never have so many athletes adopted the "as Black as you can get" baldness look, as Isaac Hayes once called it, as in the current era. Baldness is in vogue—courtesy of Michael Jordan. As David Halberstam notes: "Jordan, shaved head and all, had given America nothing less than a new definition of beauty for a new age."[14]

While part of Jordan's beauty clearly stems from his boyish good looks and classically proportioned features—he is arguably the most handsome, most photogenic and telegenic player in the history of the NBA—he is also, like his head, portrayed as the epitome of clean: clean in lifestyle—a wholesome, loving, family man with a genuine fondness for the people who matter the most, kids—"the embodiment of American virtue" as Naughton puts it;[15] clean in behavior—a welcome breath of fresh air amid the trenchant cynicism, demonic racial stereotypes, and ethical pollution that permeate contemporary professional sports;[16] and clean in body—no tattoos, no marks or blemishes, no imperfections, just a smooth, gleaming, purple-brown-hued skin—and no hair. "No white body could ever look so clean," Roger Gilbert intones.[17]

His game is clean, too. He plays "pure" basketball—no bullying, no deliberate fouling, no taunting—just technically sound offensive and defensive basketball. Although he clearly has "skills," his real genius lies in his astonishing creativity and his unrelenting competitiveness. It is the combination of talent and will, creativity and discipline, that defines Jordan as what many would characterize as the greatest player ever. His baldness epitomizes his primeval athleticism; it reduces him to a singular basketball essence. As Gilbert writes: "Removing what was left of his hair made its absence into another reflection of will, purity, purpose, not accident or entropy."[18]

Of course Jordan has had help in both the real and simulated construction of his image. Just as Prospero had his Caliban, and Los had his Urizen, so Jordan had his Rodman. As Gilbert so beautifully puts it: "While Jordan is sublime, transcendent, 'great,' Rodman is profane, immanent, 'bad.' Where Jordan is pure, clean, universal, Rodman is impure, dirty, particular. If Jordan's a hero, Rodman's an antihero; if Jordan is spirit and will, Rodman is matter and appetite."[19] Like Madonna, whom he appropriately dated, Rodman is one of the great automythologists of modern culture, whose cross-dressing, gender-bending, homoerotic, tattooed, trash-talking, "bad-as-I-wanna-be" psycho-act accentuates Jordan's textual innocence and bodily cleanliness. As if to fully consummate the juxtaposition, "the Worm" sports an ever-changing Day-Glo coiffure that features a bizarre and totally unpredictable admixture of style and color. Rodman, like his hairstyle, is theatrical, flamboyant, histrionic, a player who plays with the non-essentials, living on the sport's periphery and causing a distraction both on and off the court. Jordan, with pristine dome, is a streamlined essence, a missile purged of secondary characteristics, sleek and abstract, an ethereal player who epitomizes the essential skills and occupies a central place within the panoply of the game. Jordan rises up; Rodman gets down.[20] One is the Prince of Light and the other the Prince of Darkness.[21]

There is one more dimension to the aesthetics of Jordan's baldness—the sexual dimension. After all, he is, as bell hooks argues, "the quintessential symbol of fetishized eroticized black male body as object of spectacle."[22] But he is more than just a sex symbol—in fact the pre-eminent black athletic sex symbol—he is a phallic symbol. His sensual bald head, circumcised and protruding, shiny and moist, has made the phallic look chic among millions of young men around the world, not to mention among players in the NBA, hard bodies whose height accentuates and is indeed manipulated to celebrate phallic imagery. Even in the NBA sex sells!

But while the aesthetics and psychosexual salience of black hairstyles are not unimportant or uninteresting, the sociopolitical significance of black hair is perhaps even more engaging and compelling. Hair, or the culturally specific articulations and uses of hair as a symbol of African-American identity, has a long and fascinating history.[23] For black Americans, hair has always played a pivotal role in the politics of appearance. As Kobena Mercer notes, when race structures social relations of power, hair becomes charged with symbolic currency.[24] During the fin de siècle, for example, racial ideologies posited specific relationships between skin color, hair texture and style, and the possibilities for intelligence, social progress, and cultural legitimacy. Kinky hair, wide noses, and full lips easily translated into "ignorant," "uncivilized," and "infantile." On the other hand, the Afro hairstyles of the '60s and '70s were clearly decipherable statements about racial empowerment, brazen challenges to a traditional white aesthetic that had long rendered curly hair a significant aspect of the iconography of inferiority. In other words, the creation, production, and consumption of any particular hairstyle, whether it be Afro or dreadlocks, nappy hair or curly perm, has remained closely interwoven with ideologies of racial identity, social and political advancement, and emancipation. Responding to a critique of her film, *Daughters of the Dust*, that "it's all about hair," black filmmaker Julie Dash responded: "There's a lot of drama around Black hair...I could be a filmmaker who was myopic about it, like this really isn't an issue, but that would be untrue."[25] Because hair is subject to human management, hair style becomes a medium through which social messages and political statements can be conveyed and aesthetic standards of the dominant culture can be contested.

As part of the politics of appearance, the shaved head has retained a storied place in the history of black Americans. Eighteenth-century slaveholders resorted to head shaving as a form of punishment. According to one newspaper advertisement, Peter, a frequent runaway, had been branded "S on the cheek and R on the other" and had had his hair entirely cut off.[26] Ironically, as indentured servitude evolved into the race-based institution of slavery, escaping male slaves, seeking to convince bounty hunters that they belonged to the privileged class of free blacks, intentionally shaved their heads to eradicate the genetic evidence of their ancestry. One runaway slave, for example, was described in the *New York Weekly Journal* as a "mulatto man, aged 23, pretty fair with his head commonly shaved in order to make himself pass for a white man."[27]

More recently, close-cropped styles have been associated with the Reagan-Bush years, with their emphasis on power suits and corporate budgets. Metaphorically speaking, black men exchanged their Afro picks for wave caps and electric shavers as they went off in search of careers at prestigious law firms, financial establishments, and Fortune 500 companies. For postmodern Jordanologist David Andrews, MJ's mediated identity, created and developed primarily by Nike (with the assistance of Spike Lee's media savvy), was borne out of—and subsequently vindicated—the reactionary political climate of Reaganism. The hyperreal Air Jordan, like his mediated contemporary Heathcliff Huxtable (Bill Cosby's lead character in *The Cosby Show*)—as well as a host of other appropriated African-American entertainers including Whoopi Goldberg, Eddie Murphy, and Oprah Winfrey—became seductive simulations of the entire Reaganite project.[28] As Andrews puts it:

> By embodying the neo-liberal economics, neo-conservative politics, and moralistic cultural traditionalism of the New Right, the Nike-initiated Jordan

79

narrative celebrated Reaganism's morally corrupt and criminally negligent vision of a colorblind American society. Within this hypermythological realm, individual agency was exalted as the primary determinant of individual success, and the socially inscripted experiences and identities associated with racially based discrimination and exploitation were viewed as distant and irrelevant remnants of the past.[29]

While you may not buy the metaphor that Jordan represents the Nike-wearing, Reaganite reincarnation of Horatio Alger, it is hard not to acknowledge the fact, and the consequences of the fact, that he has become the black replicant of a white model, that he has as Gilbert puts it "effectively replaced Leonardo's famous diagrammed and encircled drawing of the ideal human figure" and "remade our image of Man, of human perfection in masculine form, substituting his own African-American body for the old European model."[30] Recognizing that Jordan has managed to be both the "downest brother" and at the same time the "whitest bread," Denzin asserts that he "is a black man who is not black";[31] or as Henry Louis Gates nuances it—Jordan's job today is to be the man behind the black man who is not really black.[32] Like the biblical Samson, although no doubt shorn even closer, Jordan has to some extent been de-racialized, certainly de-radicalized, by the very baldness that has helped transform him into one of the world's potentially most transformative political agents.

But, Jordan has repeatedly and consistently repudiated identification with any politicized notion of blackness. He has repeatedly refused to accept any responsibility for the Nike-driven exploitation of urban black youth; he has shouldered no blame in the ugly spate of urban "sneaker killings"; he chose not to lend his support to African-American Harvey Gantt in a desperately close senatorial race in Jordan's home state of North Carolina against archconservative Jesse Helms; and he responded to revelations about Third World sweatshops with the now infamous line that "Republicans buy sneakers too." Unlike many of his forebears, including Muhammad Ali, Tommie Smith, Arthur Ashe, and Harry Edwards, Jordan has neither embraced the challenges nor assumed the risks that could have transformed him into a productive and proactive force in the nation's racial drama. He has become, as black Chicago political satirist Aaron Freeman calls him, a "transcendental irrelevance."[33]

Even though I agree with Michael Dyson that Jordan's iconography has enormous subversive potential, that "his black body—graceful and powerful, elegant and dark—symbolizes the possibilities of other black bodies to remain safe long enough to survive within the limited but significant sphere of basketball,"[34] Jordan has in fact chosen to lend his image only to a visual aesthetics and economics that reaffirms a repressive, racialized body politics. As bell hooks writes:

> Rather than oppose those forms of commodification that reinvent the black male body in ways that subordinate and subjugate, today's black male athlete "submits" to any objectified use of his person that brings huge monetary reward. Black male capitulation to a neo-colonial white supremacist patriarchal commodification signals the loss of political agency, the absence of radical politics.[35]

Consequently, although Jordan has eschewed political activism and protected his image of political neutrality—"I never had an Afro, even when I was younger," Jordan once insightfully intoned[36]—he is certainly not politically neutral, even if, in Arthur Ashe's words, he may well have been "politically neutered." His politics in fact are deeply rooted in both capitalist and imperialist notions of power and influence.

And so, let me address the final dimension of his hairless Airness's hairlessness—baldness as brand. In an age of hype and hyperconsumerism—where simulation and appearance count as much as substance and authenticity, where show business often seems to be the only business, and where "image is everything," as Andre Agassi reminds us—"Brand Jordan" has been estimated by *Fortune* to have impacted the American economy to the tune of about $10 billion.[37] Because Michael Jordan transcends race, age, gender, and income, and because he has been marketed as the fusion of athletic excellence and progressive, multiracial masculinity—as David Breskin in *Gentleman's Quarterly* quips: "we may not make cars or TVs but we turn out a helluva Michael Jordan"[38]—Jordan's body has become enshrined as universal logo, a commodity sign that furthers the international ambitions of a spectacular array of corporations including Nike, Coca-Cola, McDonalds, Hanes, Bijan, MCI, Wheaties, and Gatorade. In a sense Jordan has become a new kind of global royalty, the celebrated messenger for a burgeoning global capitalism that has been resisted and critiqued as yet another form of the westernization, or even Americanization, of the planet—what LaFeber appropriately calls "the swooshification of the world."[39] The silhouetted image of Jordan's bald head hovers over the planet like a euphoric corporate hallucinogenic, packaged and hawked across the landscape of a logomaniacal culture by an aggressive corporate agenda that has fashioned a commercially viable global language of appearance and image. In interesting ways, the marketing of Jordan is emblematic of a new paradigm that conflates all distinctions between branding and culture, leaving no room for unmarked, unbranded space—including the human body.[40]

In *Interaction Ritual*, Erving Goffman argues that through rituals "societies everywhere...mobilize their members as self-regulating participants in social encounters...individuals are taught to be perceptive...to have pride, honor, and dignity...to have tact and a certain amount of poise." These traits must be built into "persons if practical use is to be made of them as interactants...it is these elements that are referred to in part when one speaks of universal human nature."[41] The problem is that the universal human nature that Jordan announces erases race—diversity sold as mono-multiculturalism, to use Naomi Klein's phrase.[42] And this, as Denzin argues, "seems to be the last requirement of a global capitalism: cultural differences disappear, to be replaced by a universal, circumspect human nature that knows its place in the order of things."[43] Is this what we want our athletes to be? Is this all that Michael Jordan's bald head really is? Just another billboard? Just another advertising space in the service of an emergent global monoculture, a monoculture driven by western and more specifically American imperialist ambitions?

1. Kobena Mercer, "Black Hair/Style Politics," in *Out There: Marginalization and Contemporary Cultures*, ed. Russell Ferguson, Martha Gever, Trinh T. Minh-ha, and Cornel West (Cambridge, Mass.: MIT Press, 1990), 248.

2. Ingrid Banks, *Hair Matters: Beauty, Power, and Black Women's Consciousness* (New York: New York University Press, 2000).

3. Harry Edwards, roundtable discussion at Saginaw Valley State University, Saginaw, Michigan.

4. John Hoberman, *Darwin's Athletes: How Sport Has Damaged Black America and Preserved the Myth of Race* (Boston: Houghton Mifflin, 1997), xiv.

5. R. Kearney, *The Wake of the Imagination: Toward a Postmodern Culture* (Minneapolis: University of Minnesota Press, 1989).

6. Milan Kundera, *Immortality* (New York: Harper Collins, 1990), 114.

7. See Michael Jordan, *Rare Air: Michael on Michael*, ed. Mark Vancil, photos by Walter Iooss (San Francisco: Collins, 1993), 111.

8. There are of course more photographs of Michael Jordan than one could possibly imagine—either with or without hair. There are also numerous photograph books on Michael Jordan. Among the best are Michael Jordan, *Rare Air* and *More Rare Air: I'm Back*, ed. Mark Vancil, photos by Walter Iooss (San Francisco: Collins, 1995); and *The Definitive Word on Michael—As Told by His Friends and Foes* (Dallas: Beckett, 1998).

9. David Halberstam, *Playing for Keeps: Michael Jordan and the World He Made* (New York: Random House, 1999), 7.

10. David Andrews, "Excavating Michael Jordan: Notes on a Critical Pedagogy of Sporting Representation," in Genvieve Rail, ed., *Sport and Postmodern Times* (Albany: State University of New York Press, 1998), 199.

11. See Henry Louis Gates, "Annals of Marketing: Net Worth," *The New Yorker*, 1 June 1998, 48–61.

12. Norman Denzin, "Representing Michael" in *Michael Jordan, Inc.: Corporate Sport, Media Culture, and Late Modern America*, ed. David L. Andrews (Albany: State University of New York Press, 2001), 3.

13. See Lorna Campbell, "Great Moments in Hair," *The Washingtonian*, August 1998, 101–102; Nelson George, "Rare Jordan," *Essence*, vol. 27, no. 7, November 1996, 106–108; Richard Mayers, "Cool Pose: Black Masculinity and Sports," in *Sport, Men, and the Gender Order:*

Critical Feminist Perspectives, ed. Michael Messner and Donald F. Sabo (Champaign, Ill.: Human Kinetics, 1990), 109–114; "They Really Want to Be Like Mike," *Los Angeles Times*, 4 June 1999, sec. E, 1.

14. David Halberstam, *Playing for Keeps*, 11.

15. Jim Naughton, *Taking to the Air: The Rise of Michael Jordan* (New York: Warner Books, 1992), 154.

16. There is no doubt that the revelations about his gambling activities and especially more recently about his marital infidelities have tarnished his image; but for most of his days in professional basketball he maintained a squeaky-clean resume. As Cleo Corporation's vice-president for marketing and development once put it: "We know Walt Disney will never allow Mickey Mouse to have a marital problem. We know Donald Duck is never going to beat Daisy. Yogi Bear is probably not going to develop a drug problem. But now we have a human being. You worry about human beings. But with Michael it is different. Michael is such a wholesome kid." Quoted in Naughton, *Taking to the Air*, 154–155.

17. Roger Gilbert, "Air, Worm, Pip, Zen: The Chicago Bulls as Sacred Book, *Salmagundi* 118–119 (Spring/Summer 1998): 251.

18. Gilbert, "Air, Worm, Pip, Zen."

19. Gilbert, "Air, Worm, Pip, Zen," 254.

20. For other juxtapositional analyses of Jordan and Rodman, see Denzin, "Representing Michael"; Gates, "Annals of Marketing: Net Worth"; and John Edgar Wideman, "Playing Dennis Rodman," *The New Yorker*, 29 April and 6 May 1996, 94–95.

21. Halberstam, *Playing for Keeps*, 349.

22. bell hooks, "Feminism Inside: Toward a Black Body Politic," in *Black: Representations of Masculinity in Contemporary American Art*, ed. Thelma Golden (New York: Harry N. Abrams, 1994), 134.

23. For historical treatments of black Americans' hair see Ayana D. Byrd and Lori L. Tharps, *Hair Story: Untangling the Roots of Black Hair in America* (New York: St. Martin's Press, 2001); Lloyd Boston, *Men of Color: Fashion, History, and Fundamentals* (New York: Artisan, 1998); Noliwe M. Rooks, *Hair Raising: Beauty, Culture, and African American Women* (New Brunswick, N.J.: Rutgers

University Press, 1996); Shane White and Graham J. White, *Stylin': African-American Expressive Culture from its Beginning to the Zoot Suit* (Ithaca: Cornell University Press, 1998).

24. Kobena Mercer, "Black Hair/Style Politics," 249.

25. Quoted in Greg Tate, "Of Homegirl Goddesses and Geechee Women," *Village Voice*, 4 June 1991, 72 and 78.

26. See Lathan A. Windley, comp., *Runaway Slave Advertisements: A Documentary History from the 1730s to 1790*, vol. 1 (Westport, Conn.: Greenwood, 1983), 311.

27. Quoted in Byrd and Tharps, *Hair Story*, 18.

28. David Andrews, "The Fact(s) of Michael Jordan's Blackness: Excavating a Floating Racial Signifier," in David Andrews ed., *Michael Jordan, Inc.*, 115.

29. Andrews, "Excavating Michael Jordan," 200.

30. Gilbert, "Air, Worm, Pip, Zen," 250–251.

31. Denzin, "Representing Michael," 6.

32. Gates, "Annals of Marketing: Net Worth," 60.

33. Quoted in Naughton, *Taking to the Air*, 206.

34. Michael Dyson, "Be Like Mike?" in Michael Dyson, ed., *Reflecting Black: African-American Cultural Criticism* (Minneapolis: University of Minnesota Press, 1993), 74.

35. bell hooks, "Feminism Inside," 133.

36. Quoted in Bob Greene, *Hang Time: Days and Dreams with Michael Jordan* (New York: Doubleday, 1992), 133.

37. See Roy S. Johnson, "The Jordan Effect: The World's Greatest Basketball Player is also One of its Greatest Brands. What is his Impact on the Economy?" *Fortune*, 22 June 1998, 124–126, 130–132, and 134–136.

38. David Breskin, "On Michael," *Gentleman's Quarterly*, December 1989, 8.

39. W. LaFeber, *Michael Jordan and the New Global Capitalism* (New York: W.W. Norton, 1999), 189.

40. I am thinking here of athletes, especially boxers and wrestlers, whose exposed bodies are tattooed with commercials, advertisements, and promotions, as well as athletes who fashion commercial logos and symbols into their hairstyles.

41. Erving Goffman, *Interaction Ritual* (New York: Doubleday, 1976).

42. Naomi Klein, *No Logo* (New York: Picador, 1999), 116.

43. Denzin, "Representing Michael," 11.

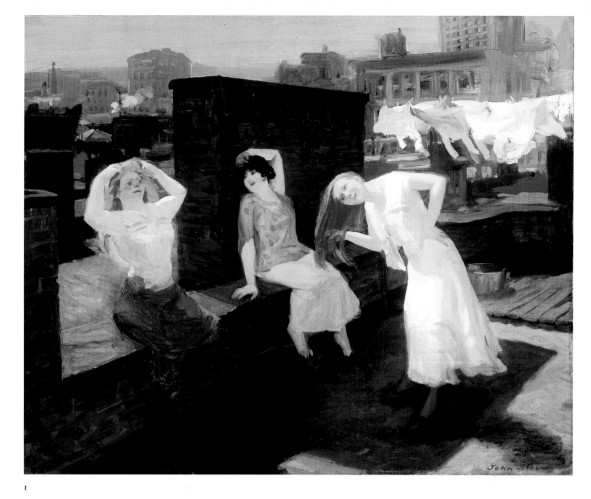

1

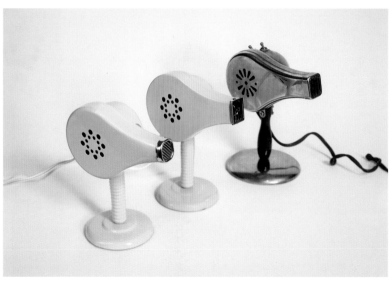

2

PLATE 1
John Sloan
*Sunday, Women Drying Their
Hair*, 1912
Oil on canvas
26 1/8 x 32 1/8 inches

PLATE 2
Electric hair dryers, 20th century
Approx. 9 1/2 x 7 1/4 x 4 1/2 inches
each

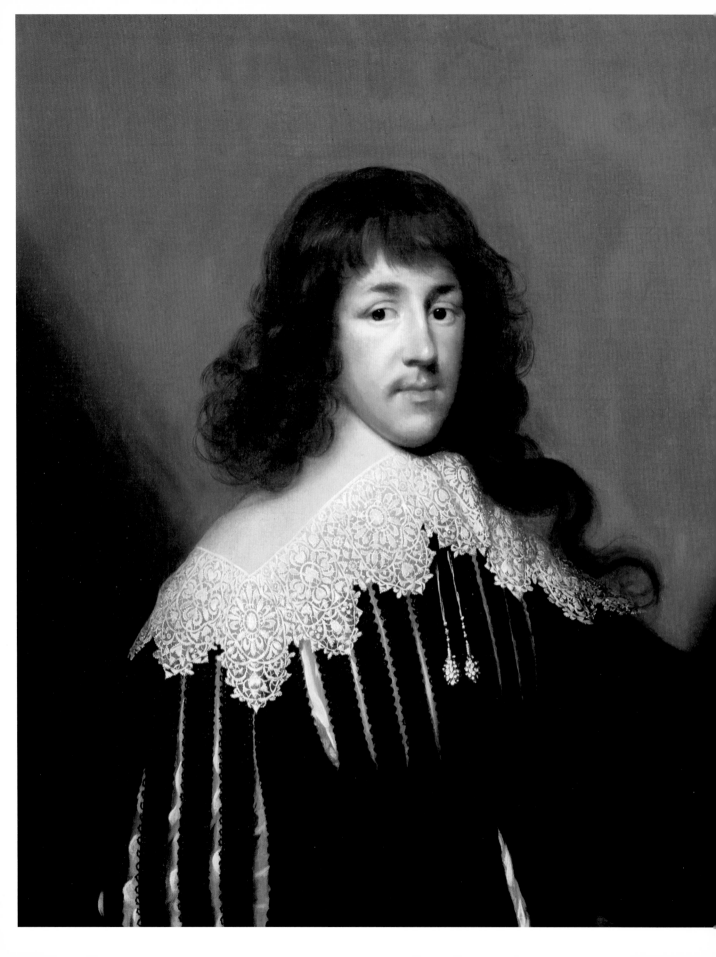

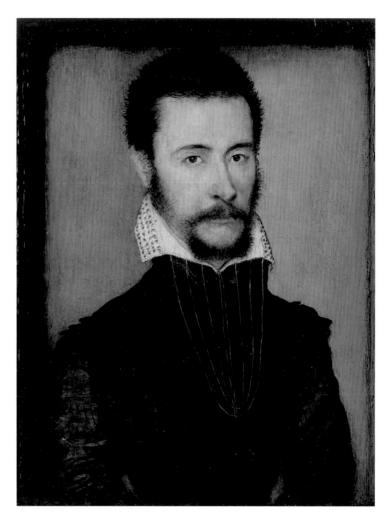

4

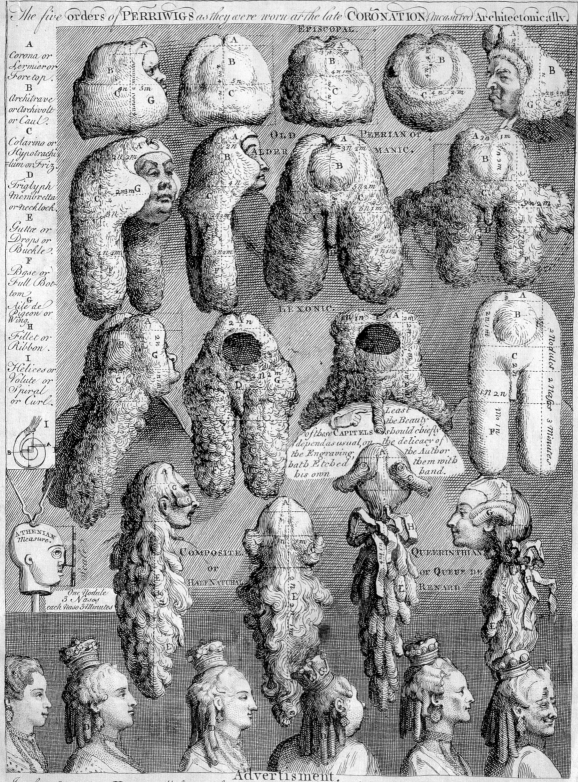

The five orders of PERRIWIGS as they were worn at the late CORONATION measured Architectonically.

EPISCOPAL.

OLD ALDER PEERIAN OR MANIC.

LEXONIC.

COMPOSITE. OR HALF NATURAL.

QUEERINTHIAN. OR QUEUE DE RENARD.

A Corona or Lermier or Foretop.
B Architrave or Archivolt or Caul.
C Colarino or Hypotrachilium or Friz.
D Triglyph Membretta or Necklock.
E Guttæ or Drops or Buckle.
F Base or Full Bottom.
G Aile de Pigeon or Wing.
H Fillet or Ribbon.
I Hélices or Volute or Spiral or Curl.

ATHENIAN Measure.
One Nodule 3 Nasos each Naso 34 Minutes

Least the Beauty of these CAPITELS should chiefly depend as usual, on the delicacy of the Engraving, the Author hath Etched them with his own hand.

Advertisment.

In about Seventeen Years will be compleated, in Six Volums, folio, price, Fifteen Guineas, the exact measurements of the PERRIWIGS of the ancients; taken from the Statues, Bustos & Baso-Relievos of Athens, Palmira, Balbec, and Rome, by MODESTO Perriwig-meter from Lagado.
NB. None will be Sold but to Subscribers. —— Publish'd as the Act directs Oct. 15. 1761 by W. Hogarth.

5

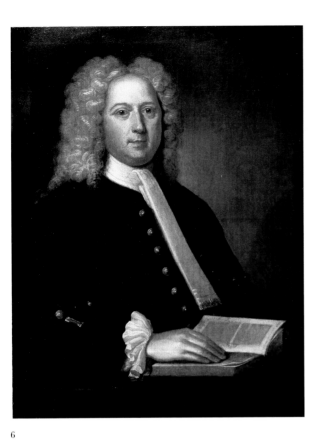

6

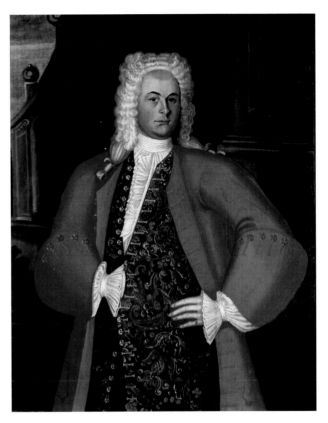

7

PLATE 5

William Hogarth

The Five Orders of Periwigs, 1761

Etching and engraving

12 1/4 x 9 inches

PLATE 6

John Smibert

William Lambert, 1734

Oil on canvas

35 7/8 x 28 1/8 inches

PLATE 7

Attributed to John Heaten

Jeremias Van Rensselaer, c. 1745

Oil on canvas

48 x 39 inches

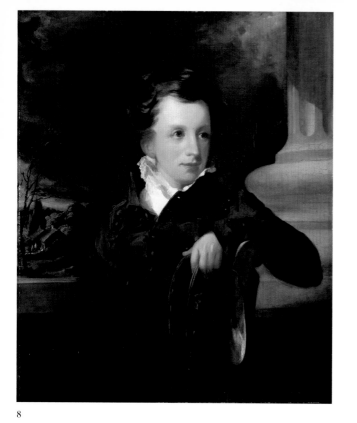

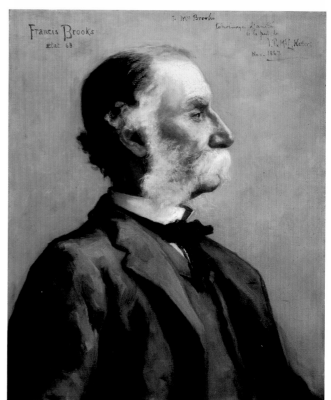

8

9

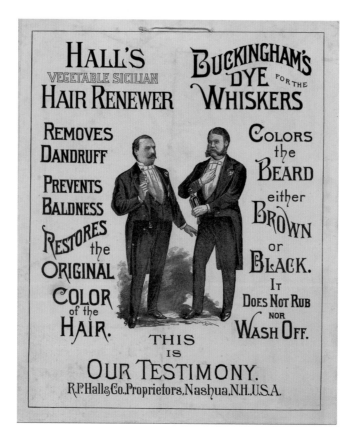

10

PLATE 8
Thomas Sully
Tom Wharton, 1800–10
Oil on canvas
30 1/8 x 25 1/8 inches

PLATE 9
J.P. Mc L. Watters
Francis Brooks., 1887
Oil on canvas
24 x 20 inches

PLATE 10
Hall's Hair Renewer and
Buckingham's Dye
Advertisement
14 x 11 1/2 inches

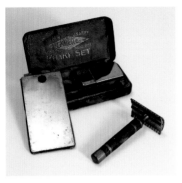

11

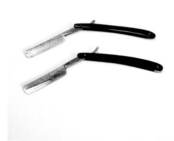

12

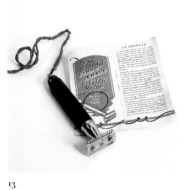

13

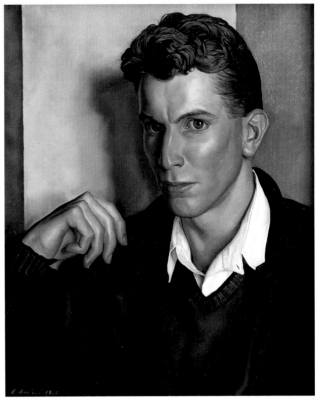

15

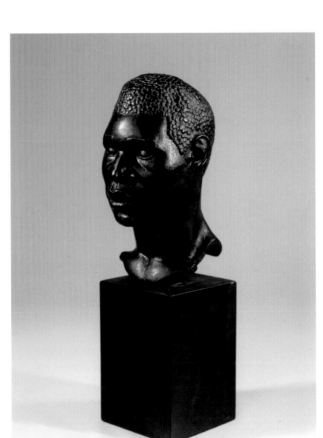

14

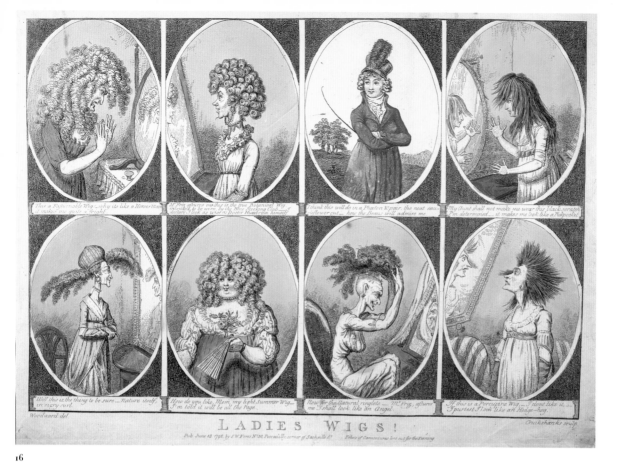

16

PLATE 16
Isaac Cruikshank
Ladies Wigs!, 1798
Hand-colored etching
14 3/8 x 19 1/2 inches

PLATE 17
Published by William Humphrey
Beauty's Lot, n.d.
Engraving
12 3/4 x 7 7/8 inches

PLATE 18
Published by Matthew and Mary Darly
*Oh Heigh Oh – Or a View of the
Back Settlements*, 1776
Engraving
13 7/8 x 9 7/8 inches

PLATE 19
Anonymous
*Mlle. des Faveurs à la Promenade
à Londres*, 18th century
Hand-colored etching
13 1/2 x 10 inches

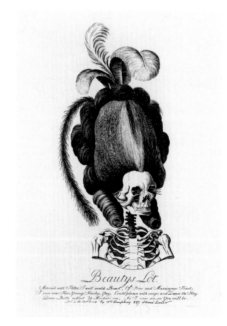

17

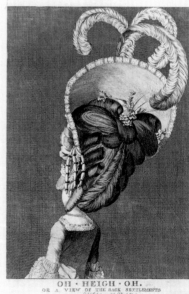

18

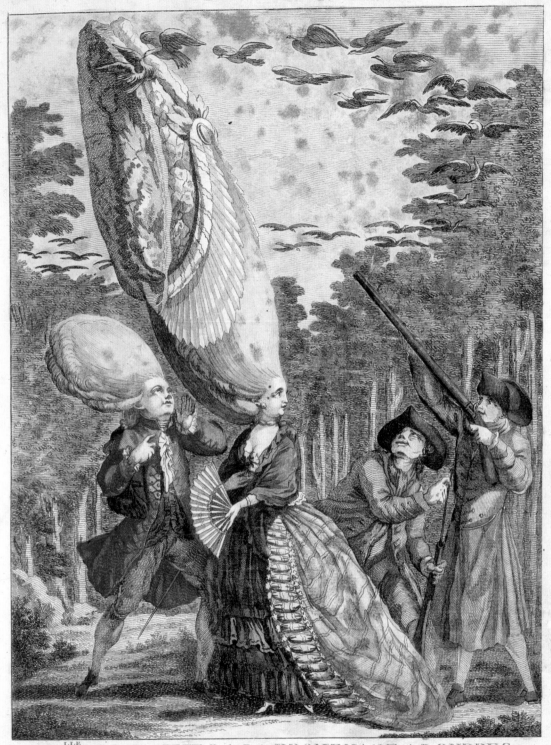

MLLE DES FAVEURS A LA PROMENADE A LONDRES

Ma Coëffure en effet reſſemble au Colombier ;   Mais en tirant deſſus Anglois qu'allez vous faire ;
Puisque tous ces Pigeons viennent s'y repoſer.   Faut-il pour nos Folies, vous rendre téméraires.

19

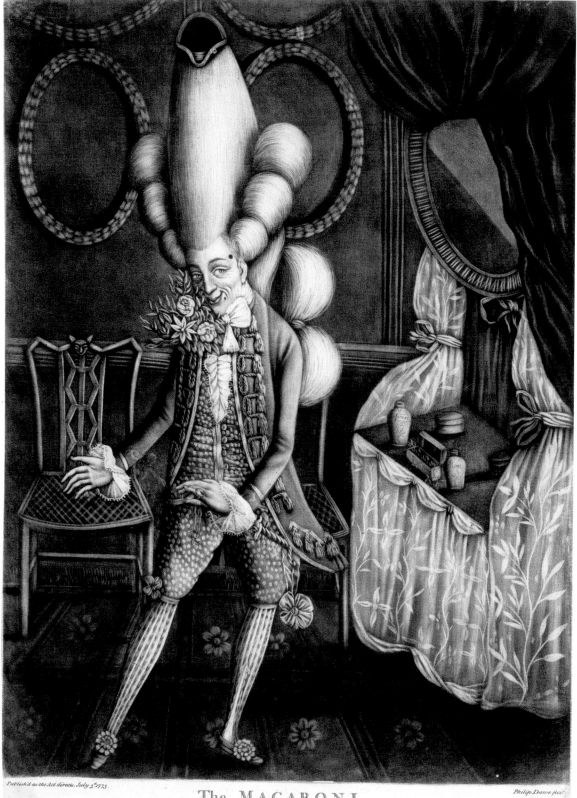

Publish'd as the Act directs, July 3.ᵈ 1773.

The MACARONI.
A real Character at the late Masquerade.

Printed for John Bowles, at Nᵒ 13 in Cornhill.

Philip Dawe fecit

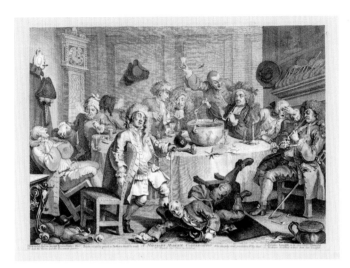

PLATE 20

Philip Dawe

The Macaroni. A Real Character at the
Late Masquerade, 1773

Mezzotint

13 7/8 x 10 inches

PLATE 21

William Hogarth

A Midnight Modern Conversation,
1732–33

Etching and engraving

13 1/2 x 18 5/8 inches

PLATE 22

Published by R. Sayer & J. Bennett

What Is This My Son Tom, 1774

Mezzotint

13 7/8 x 9 7/8 inches

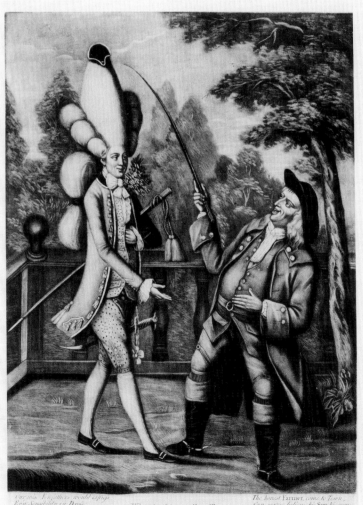

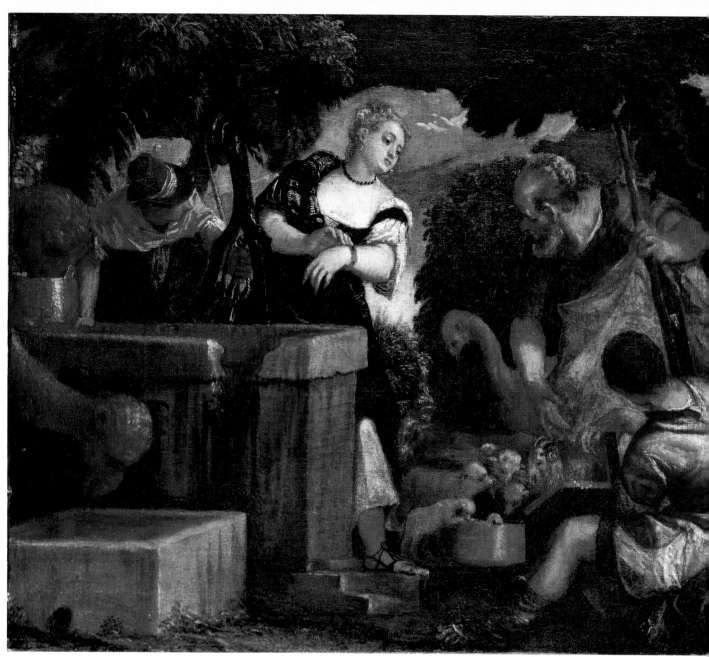

23

PLATE 23

Paolo Caliari Veronese

Rebecca at the Well, c. 1570

Oil on canvas

18 1/2 x 22 inches

PLATE 24

John Hesselius

Eleanor Addison, c. 1773–75

Oil on canvas

30 1/8 x 25 1/8 inches

PLATE 25

James Peale

Jane Ramsey Peale, c. 1802

Oil on canvas

28 1/8 x 20 7/8 inches

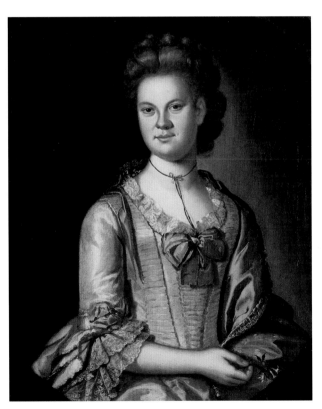

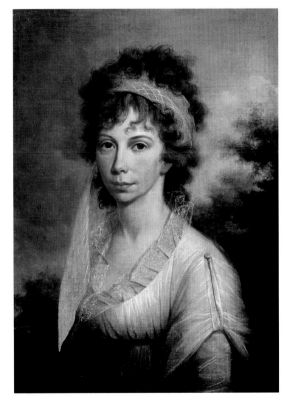

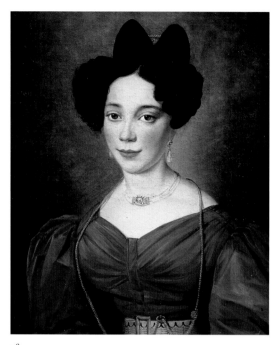

26

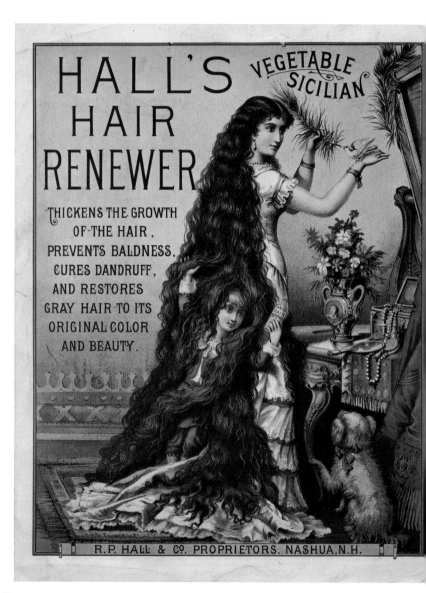

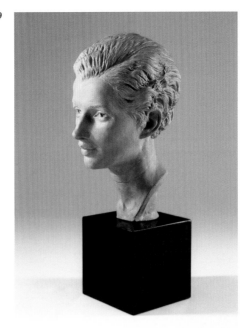

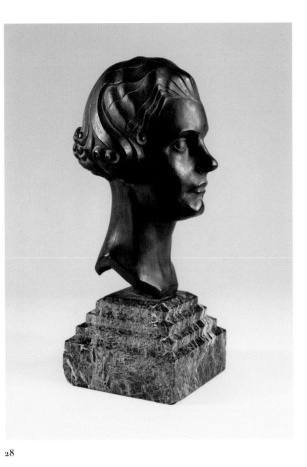

PLATE 26
Anonymous, French
Lady with Giraffe-Inspired Hair Style, c. 1830
Oil on canvas
24 x 19 5/8 inches

PLATE 27
Hall's Hair Renewer
Advertisement
13 7/8 x 11 inches

PLATE 28
Wheeler Williams
Portrait of Sylvia, 1923
Bronze
12 3/4 x 7 1/2 x 7 3/4 inches

PLATE 29
Edward McCartan
Portrait of a Young Woman, 1934
Terracotta
11 3/4 x 6 1/2 x 7 inches

PLATE 30
Wig of Celia Cruz, c. 1980
13 x 11 x 11 inches

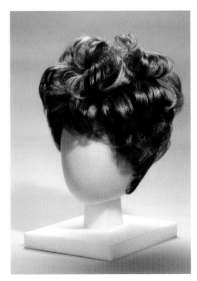

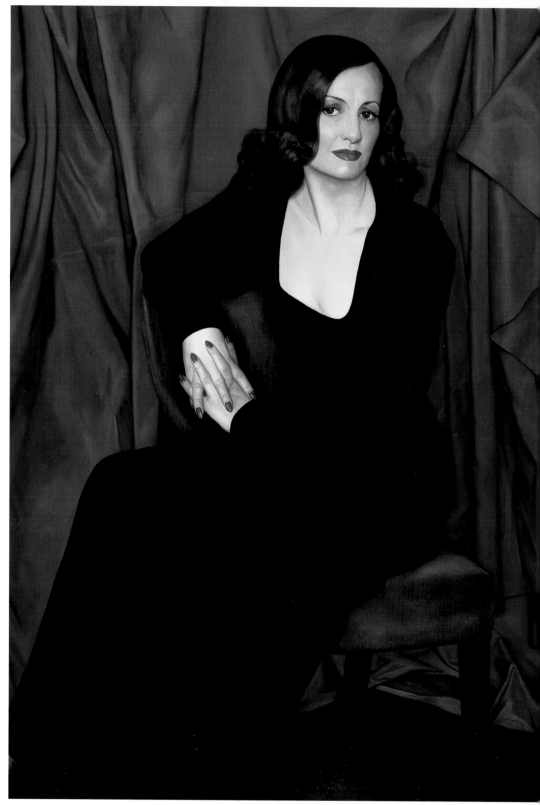

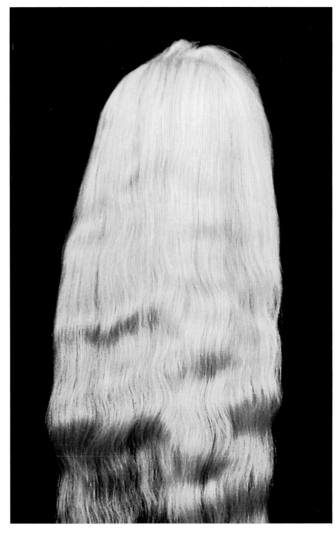

33

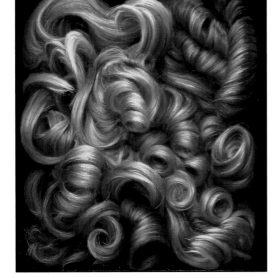

32

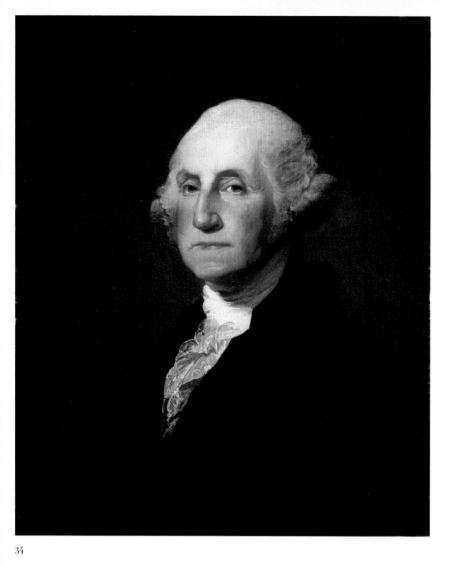

34

PLATE 34

Gilbert Stuart

George Washington, after 1796

Oil on canvas

26 1/2 x 21 1/2 inches

PLATES 35–37

Compiled by Leigh Hunt

Hair of Famous Writers

(**Mary Shelley**, Pl. 35;

Elizabeth Barrett Browning, Pl. 36;

Robert Browning, Pl. 37)

Human hair and prints

Each page 14 1/2 x 10 3/4 inches

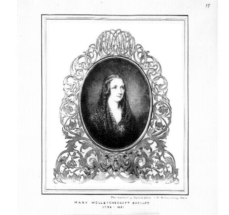

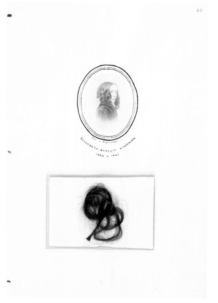

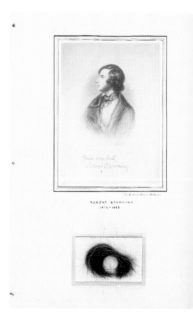

35   36   37

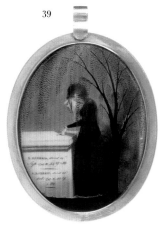

39

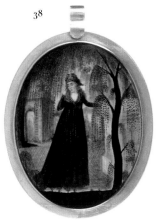

38

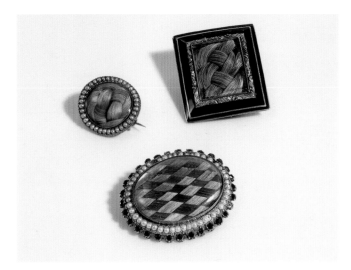

40

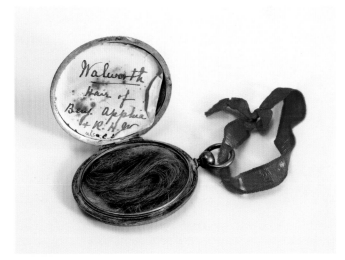

41

PLATE 38

possibly by Ezra Ames

Ludlow Mourning Locket, c. 1800

Watercolor on ivory, human hair,
gold case

3 3/8 x 2 3/8 inches

PLATE 39

possibly by Ezra Ames

Egberts Mourning Locket, c. 1800

Watercolor on ivory, human hair,
gold case

3 1/2 x 2 3/8 inches

PLATE 40

Mourning jewelry

Human hair, metal, and stones

Approx. 1 x 1 inch each

PLATE 41

**Mourning Locket (with hair of
Chancellor Walworth, his parents,
and son)**

Human hair and silver

3 1/8 x 2 inches

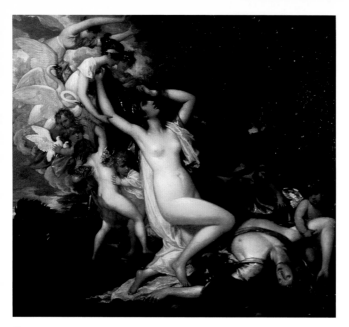

42

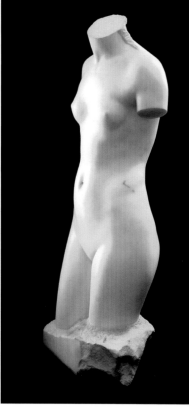

44

PLATE 42
Benjamin West
Venus Lamenting Adonis, 1803
Oil on panel
15 1/2 x 16 3/4 inches

PLATE 43
Birgit Dieker
Beasty Girl, 2001
Human hair, lamb's wool,
glass eyes, epoxy
70 x 24 x 12 inches

PLATE 44
Mario J. Korbel
Female Torso, 1927
Marble
39 x 15 3/4 x 9 5/8 inches

PLATE 45
Edward Kienholz
Bunny, Bunny, You're So Funny, 1962
Mixed media
31 1/2 x 33 x 12 1/2 inches

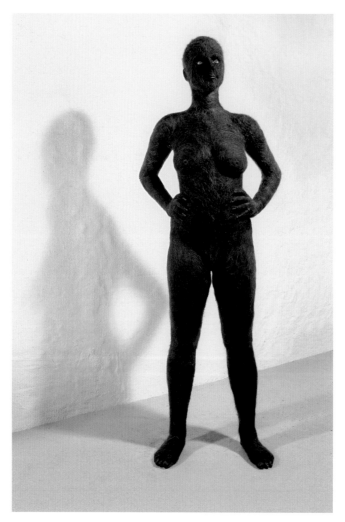

43

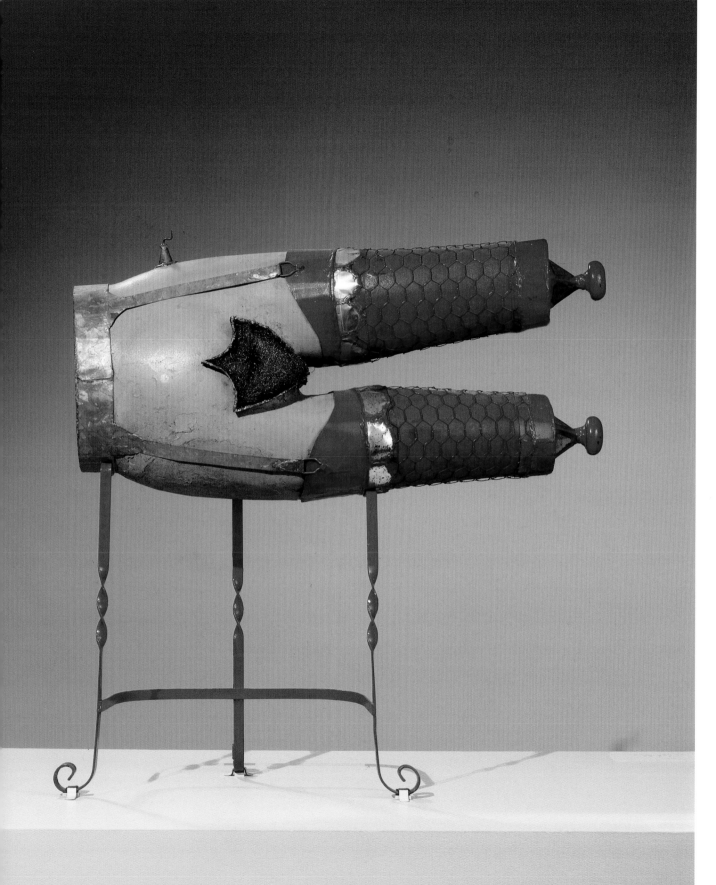

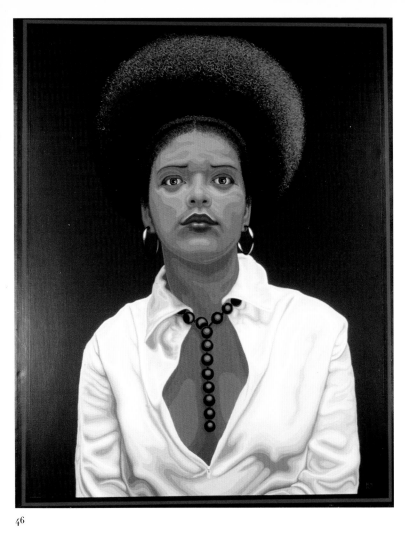

46

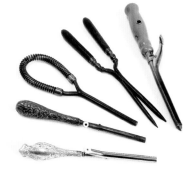

47

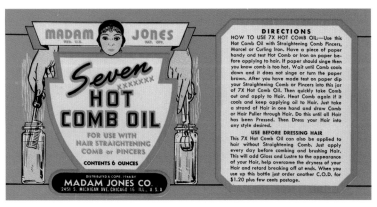

48

PLATE 46

H. Lee Hirsche

Blue Necklace, 1973

Acrylic on canvas

60 x 48 inches

PLATE 47

Crimpers

Approx. 8 x 1 x 3 inches each

PLATE 48

Curling irons

Approx. 8 x 1 x 1 inches each

PLATE 49

Madam Jones Seven X Hot Comb Oil

Advertisement

3 3/4 x 7 1/8 inches

49

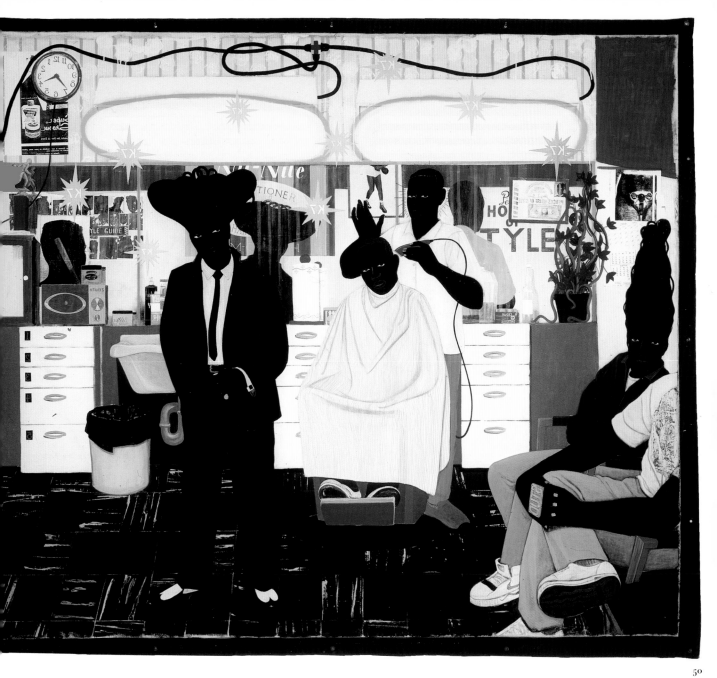

PLATE 50

Kerry James Marshall

De Style, 1993

Acrylic and collage on canvas

104 x 122 inches

PLATE 51

Wig of Bozo the Clown, c. 1960

4 1/2 x 27 1/2 x 17 inches

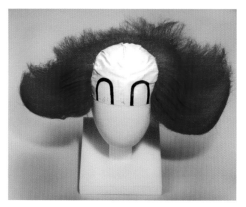

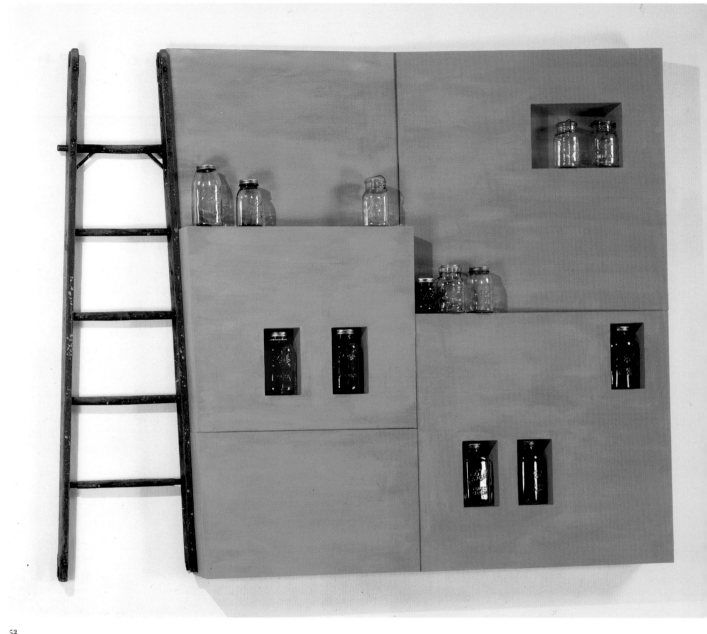

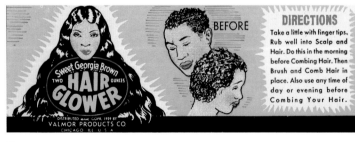

PLATE 52

Debra Priestly

Lookin Glass #4, 1999

Mixed media on birch

76 x 96 x 6 inches

PLATE 53

Sweet Georgia Brown Hair Glower

Advertisement

1 5/8 x 6 1/8 inches

CONTRIBUTORS

GERALD M. ERCHAK received his Ph.D. in social anthropology from Harvard University in 1976, and in the same year joined the faculty of Skidmore College, where he is now Professor of Anthropology. He is the author of *The Anthropology of Self and Behavior* (Rutgers University Press, 1992) and numerous articles in the field of psychological anthropology. He has carried out field research in Liberia, Micronesia, South Africa, and, most recently, Brazil.

PENNY HOWELL JOLLY is Professor of Art History and William R. Kenan Chair of Liberal Arts at Skidmore College. She has published articles on Flemish and Italian artists in the *Art Bulletin*, *Burlington Magazine*, and elsewhere, and is the author of *Made in God's Image? Eve and Adam in the Genesis Mosaics at San Marco, Venice* (Berkeley: University of California Press, 1997).

AMELIA RAUSER is Associate Professor of Art History at Franklin and Marshall College. She has published on eighteenth-century British political prints in *Oxford Art Journal*, *Eighteenth Century Studies*, and elsewhere, and is currently at work on a book-length study of the relationship between the rise of caricature and the modern self.

JEFFREY O. SEGRAVE is Professor of Exercise Science at Skidmore College, where he has taught for twenty-five years. Currently the Director of Athletics, he has also served as the women's tennis coach and chair of the Department of Exercise Science, Dance, and Athletics. His main areas of scholarly interest are the sociology and history of sport, and he has written most extensively on the Olympic Games, women and sport, and language and sport.

SUSAN WALZER is Associate Professor of Sociology and currently chair of the Department of Sociology, Anthropology, and Social Work at Skidmore College. A former therapist and consultant, her research and teaching interests include the sociology of families and gender as well as social psychology. She is author of the book *Thinking about the Baby: Gender and Transitions into Parenthood*, as well as a number of articles about family changes and interactions.

SELECTED BIBLIOGRAPHY

Adams, Russell B., Jr. *King C. Gillette: The Man and His Wonderful Shaving Device*. Boston: Little, Brown and Co., 1978.

Banks, Ingrid. *Hair Matters: Beauty, Power, and Black Women's Consciousness*. New York: New York University Press, 2000.

Bartlett, Robert. "Symbolic Meanings of Hair in the Middle Ages." *Transactions of the Royal Historical Society* ser. 6, vol. 4 (1994): 43–60.

Basow, Susan A. "The Hairless Ideal: Women and Their Body Hair." *Psychology of Women Quarterly* 15 (1991): 83–96.

———, and Amie C. Braman. "Women and Body Hair: Social Perceptions and Attitudes." *Psychology of Women Quarterly* 22 (1998): 637–645.

Boston, Lloyd. *Men of Color: Fashion, History, Fundamentals*. New York: Artisan, 1998.

Bryer, Robin. *The History of Hair*. London: Philip Wilson Publications, 2000.

Bundles, A'Lelia Perry. *On Her Own Ground: The Life and Times of Madam C. J. Walker*. New York: Scribner, 2001.

Byrd, Ayana D., and Lori L. Tharps. *Hair Story: Untangling the Roots of Black Hair in America*. New York: St. Martin's Press, 2001.

Cash, Thomas F. "The Psychological Consequences of Androgenetic Alopecia: A Review of the Research Literature." *British Journal of Dermatology* 141 (1999): 398–405.

Clayson, Dennis E., and Micol R. C. Maughan. "Redheads and Blonds: Stereotypic Images." *Psychological Reports* 59 (1986): 811–816.

Conrad, Barnaby. *The Blonde*. San Francisco: Chronicle Books, 1999.

Cooper, Wendy. *Hair: Sex, Society, Symbolism*. New York: Stein and Day, 1971.

Corson, Richard. *Fashions in Hair: The First Five Thousand Years*. London: Peter Owen, 1971.

David, Larry. "Kiss My Head." *Men's Fashions of the Times Magazine*, 19 March 2001, 108.

Deutsch, Davida T. "Jewelry for Mourning, Love, and Fancy, 1770–1830." *Magazine Antiques* 155 (1999): 566–575.

Fisher, Will. "The Renaissance Beard: Masculinity in Early Modern England." *Renaissance Quarterly* 54 (2001): 155–185.

Gerbod, Paul. *Histoire de la Coiffure et des Coiffeurs*. Paris: Larousse, 1995.

Giacometti, Luigi. "Facts, Legends, and Myths about the Scalp throughout History." *Archives of Dermatology* 95 (1967): 629–631.

Gitter, Elisabeth G. "The Power of Women's Hair in the Victorian Imagination." *PMLA* 99 (1984): 936–954.

Grayson, Deborah R. "Is it Fake?: Black Women's Hair as Spectacle and Spec(tac)ular." *Camera Obscura* 36 (1995): 13–30.

Harris, Juliette, and Pamela Johnson, eds. *Tenderheaded: A Comb-Bending Collection of Hair Stories*. New York: Pocket Books, 2001.

Hollander, Anne. *Seeing through Clothes*. Berkeley: University of California Press, 1978.

Hope, Christine. "Caucasian Female Body Hair and American Culture." *Journal of American Culture* 5 (1982): 93–99.

Jones, Lisa. *Bulletproof Diva: Tales of Race, Sex, and Hair*. New York: Doubleday, 1994.

Lewis, J. M. "Caucasian Body Hair Management: A Key to Gender and Species Identification in U. S. Culture?" *Journal of American Culture* 10 (1987): 7–14.

Manca, Joseph. "Blond Hair as a Mark of Nobility in Ferrarese Portraiture of the Quattrocento." *Musei Ferraresi* 17 (1990/1991): 51–60.

McFadden, David R. *Hair*. New York: Cooper-Hewitt Museum, 1980.

Mellinkoff, Ruth. "Judas's Red Hair and the Jews." *Journal of Jewish Art* 9 (1982): 31–46.

Mercer, Kobena. "Black Hair/Style Politics." In *Out There: Marginalization and Contemporary Cultures*, edited by Russell Ferguson, Martha Gever, Trinh T. Minh-ha, and Cornel West, 247–264. Cambridge, Mass.: MIT Press, 1990.

Navarro, Irene G. "Hairwork of the Nineteenth Century." *Magazine Antiques* 159 (2001): 484–493.

Ogle, Robert R., Jr., and Michelle J. Fox. *Atlas of Human Hair: Microscopic Characteristics*. Boca Raton, London, New York: CRC Press, 1999.

Pitman, Joanna. *On Blondes*. London: Bloomsbury, 2003.

Pointon, Marcia. "The Case of the Dirty Beau: Symmetry, Disorder and the Politics of Masculinity." In *The Body Imaged: The Human Form and Visual Culture Since the Renaissance*, edited by Kathleen Adler and Marcia Pointon, 175–189. Cambridge: Cambridge University Press, 1993.

Retallack, G. Bruce. "Razors, Shaving and Gender Construction: An Inquiry into the Material Culture of Shaving." *Material History* Review 49 (1999): 4–19.

Rich, Melissa K., and Thomas F. Cash. "The American Image of Beauty: Media Representations of Hair Color for Four Decades." *Sex Roles* 29 (1993): 113–124.

Roberts, Mary L. "Samson and Delilah Revisited: The Politics of Women's Fashion in 1920s France." *The American Historical Review* 98 (1993): 657–684.

Robinson, Dwight E. "Fashions in Shaving and Trimming of the Beard: The Men of the *Illustrated London News*, 1842–1972." *American Journal of Sociology* 81 (1976): 1133–1141.

Rooks, Noliwe M. *Hair Raising: Beauty, Culture, and African American Women*. New Brunswick, N.J.: Rutgers University Press, 1996.

Severn, Bill. *The Long and Short of It: Five Thousand Years of Fun and Fury over Hair*. New York: McKay Co., 1971.

Trasko, Mary. *Daring Do's: A History of Extraordinary Hair*. Paris and New York: Flammarion, 1994.

Weitz, Rose. "Women and Their Hair: Seeking Power through Resistance and Accommodation." *Gender and Society* 15 (2001): 667–686.

White, Shane, and Graham J. White. "Slave Hair and African-American Culture in the Eighteenth and Nineteenth Centuries." *Journal of Southern History* 61 (1995): 45–76.

_____. *Stylin': African-American Expressive Culture from its Beginning to the Zoot Suit*. Ithaca: Cornell University Press, 1998.

Wilson, Judith. "Beauty Rites: Towards an Anatomy of Culture in African American Women's Art." *The International Review of African American Art* 11.3 (1994): 11–55.

CHECKLIST
Dimensions in inches, height x width x depth

PAINTINGS

Attributed to **CORNEILLE DE LYON**
Portrait of the Count d'Angoulême,
c. 1560
Oil on wood panel
8 1/4 x 6 1/4 inches
The Hyde Collection, Glens Falls,
New York, 1971.14

PAOLO CALIARI VERONESE
Rebecca at the Well, c. 1570
Oil on canvas
18 1/2 x 22 inches
The Hyde Collection, Glens Falls,
New York, 1971.57

CORNELIUS JOHNSON
*Portrait of a Man, probably Sir Francis
Godolphin*, 1633
Oil on canvas
31 x 24 1/2 inches
Yale Center for British Art, Paul
Mellon Collection, B1973.1.28

JOHN SMIBERT
William Lambert, 1734
Oil on canvas
35 7/8 x 28 1/8 inches
Addison Gallery of American Art,
Phillips Academy, Andover,
Massachusetts, museum purchase,
1958.55

Attributed to **JOHN HEATEN**
Jeremias Van Rensselaer, c. 1745
Oil on canvas
48 x 39 inches
Albany Institute of History & Art,
Albany, New York, Gift of Mrs.
Ledyard Cogswell, Jr., 1972.59.1

JOHN HESSELIUS
Eleanor Addison, c. 1773–75
Oil on canvas
30 1/8 x 25 1/8 inches
Addison Gallery of American Art,
Phillips Academy, Andover,
Massachusetts, gift of Mrs.
Cornelius N. Bliss, 1944.78

ADOLPH U. WERTMULLER
Edmond Charles Genet, 1784
Oil on canvas
26 x 21 3/8 inches
Albany Institute of History & Art,
bequest of Nancy Fuller Genet,
1978.6.1

GILBERT STUART
George Washington, after 1796
Oil on canvas
26 1/2 x 21 1/2 inches
Sterling and Francine Clark Art
Institute, Williamstown,
Massachusetts, 1955.16

THOMAS SULLY
Tom Wharton, 1800–10
Oil on canvas
30 1/8 x 25 1/8 inches
Addison Gallery of American Art,
Phillips Academy, Andover,
Massachusetts, museum purchase,
1969.15

JAMES PEALE
Jane Ramsey Peale, c. 1802
Oil on canvas
28 1/8 x 20 7/8 inches
Addison Gallery of American Art,
Phillips Academy, Andover,
Massachusetts, gift of the Collection
of Waldron P. Belknap. Jr., 1958.57

BENJAMIN WEST
Venus Lamenting Adonis, 1803
Oil on panel
15 1/2 x 16 3/4 inches
Jane Voorhees Zimmerli Art Museum
Rutgers, the State University of New
Jersey, ZAM purchase

EZRA AMES
Edmond Charles Genet, c. 1809–10
Oil on wood panel
30 1/8 x 23 inches
Albany Institute of History & Art,
Bequest of George Clinton Genet,
1909.21

ANONYMOUS, FRENCH
Lady with Giraffe-Inspired Hair Style,
c. 1830
Oil on canvas
24 x 19 5/8 inches
Collection of Alfred L. Chatelain and
Nancy L. Rudick

ANONYMOUS, FRENCH
Portrait of Mme. De Lapeyriere,
c. 1830
Oil on canvas
9 x 7 1/2 inches
Collection of Alfred L. Chatelain and
Nancy L. Rudick

Attributed to **FRANCES ALEXANDER**
Laura Spencer Townsend, c. 1840
Oil on canvas
30 x 25 inches
Collection of Henry Peltz,
Courtesy of the Albany Institute of
History & Art

CHARLES LORING ELLIOTT

Erastus Corning, Jr., 1864
Oil on canvas
27 x 22 inches
Albany Institute of History & Art,
Gift of Mr. and Mrs. Francis W.
Rawle, Jr., 1981.6

Governor Reuben Fenton, 1866
Oil on canvas
52 5/8 x 40 inches
Albany Institute of History & Art,
Permanent Deposit by the City of
Albany, 1971.12.9

J.P. Mc L. WATTERS

Francis Brooks, 1887
Oil on canvas
24 x 20 inches
Museum of Fine Arts, Boston A.
Shuman Collection, 1982.324

JOHN SLOAN

Sunday, Women Drying Their Hair,
1912
Oil on canvas
26 1/8 x 32 1/8 inches
Addison Gallery of American Art,
Phillips Academy, Andover,
Massachusetts, museum purchase,
1938.67

GEORGE GROSZ

Portrait of a Lady (On the Subway),
1933
Watercolor on wove paper
26 3/8 x 19 inches
Addison Gallery of American Art,
Phillips Academy, Andover,
Massachusetts, gift of Lilian and
Peter Grosz (PA 1945) in
memory of Michael Grosz (PA 1974),
1992.24

LUIGI LUCIONI

Portrait of a Young Man, 1933
Oil on canvas
22 x 18 inches
Courtesy of James Graham & Sons,
New York

Milli Monti, 1941
Oil on canvas
49 1/2 x 33 inches
Courtesy of James Graham & Sons,
New York

CHARLES SHELDON

Breck Girl (Roma Whitney), 1937
Oil on panel
43 x 32 inches
National Museum of American
History, Behring Center, Smithsonian
Institution

H. LEE HIRSCHE

Blue Necklace, 1973
Acrylic on canvas
60 x 48 inches
Collection of Lori Gladstone

FRANKLIN ALEXANDER

Mara's Morning, 1973
Oil on canvas
59 x 48 1/8 inches
Albany Institute of History & Art,
Bequest of Catherine H. Campbell,
1989.24

KERRY JAMES MARSHALL

De Style, 1993
Acrylic and collage on canvas
104 x 122 inches
Los Angeles County Museum of Art,
Purchased with funds provided by
Ruth and Jacob Bloom

RUTH MARTEN

Fire, 2002
Egg tempera on wood
13 3/4 x 14 1/2 inches
Collection of Tressa Melaura Love,
New York

Ogun, 2002
Egg tempera on wood
10 1/2 x 9 1/2 inches
Collection of Roger P. Thomas

Muscle, 2003
Egg tempera on wood
12 1/2 x 9 1/2 inches
Courtesy of the artist and Adam
Baumgold Gallery

Time II, 2003
Egg tempera on wood
11 1/2 x 15 1/2 inches
Courtesy of the artist and Adam
Baumgold Gallery

SCULPTURE

Human Hair Wreaths, late 19th
century
Hair, gilded wood frame
Dimensions variable
New York State Museum, Albany,
New York

WHEELER WILLIAMS

Portrait of Sylvia, 1923
Bronze
12 3/4 x 7 1/2 x 7 3/4 inches
Courtesy of James Graham & Sons,
New York

Head of a Black Man, 1924
Bronze
8 1/16 x 4 1/8 x 5 1/16 inches
Courtesy of James Graham & Sons,
New York

MARIO J. KORBEL
Female Torso, 1927
Marble
39 x 15 3/4 x 9 5/8 inches
Courtesy of James Graham & Sons,
New York

EDWARD McCARTAN
Portrait of a Young Woman, 1934
Terracotta
11 3/4 x 6 1/2 x 7 inches
Courtesy of James Graham & Sons,
New York

EDWARD KIENHOLZ
Bunny, Bunny, You're So Funny, 1962
Mixed media
31 1/2 x 33 x 12 1/2 inches
Williams College Museum of Art, Gift
of Susan W. and Stephen D. Paine,
Class of 1954, 85.44

MILLIE WILSON
Museum of Lesbian Dreams, 1990
Mixed media
Dimensions variable
On extended loan to the Tang Teaching
Museum from a private collection

DEBRA PRIESTLY
Lookin Glass #4, 1999
Mixed media on birch
76 x 96 x 6 inches
Collection of the artist

BIRGIT DIEKER
Beasty Girl, 2001
Human hair, lamb's wool, glass
eyes, epoxy
70 x 24 x 12 inches
Collection of Susan Crossley and
Timothy Collins

JEWELRY

Mourning Brooch, c. 1790
Human hair, gold
2 1/4 x 1 7/8 inches
Albany Institute of History & Art,
U1978.253

possibly by **EZRA AMES**
Ludlow Mourning Locket, c. 1800
Watercolor on ivory, human hair,
gold case
3 3/8 x 2 3/8 inches
Albany Institute of History & Art,
Purchase, 1973.41

Egberts Mourning Locket, c. 1800
Watercolor on ivory, human hair,
gold case
3 1/2 x 2 3/8 inches
Albany Institute of History & Art,
Gift of the estate of Miss Evelyn
Newman, 1964.31.50

Brooch, c. 1840s
Human hair, mother of pearl, gold
1 7/8 x 1 1/2 inches
Albany Institute of History & Art,
U1978.256

LE MONNIER & CIE, PARIS
Bracelet, c. 1860s
Human hair, gold
1 1/8 x 7 5/8 inches
Albany Institute of History & Art, Gift
of Mary De Camp Banks Moore,
1972.81.10

Two pins, 19th century
Human hair, metal, and stones
1 x 1 inches each
Collection of Beverley Armsden
Daniel

COLLINGWOOD & CO.
Gold tie pin, 1883
3 x 1 inches
Gernsheim Collection, Harry Ransom
Center, University of Texas-Austin

Collection of hair jewelry, 19th century
Dimensions variable
New York State Museum, Albany,
New York

Collection of hair jewelry, 19th century
Dimensions variable
Historical Society of Saratoga
Springs, Saratoga Springs, New York

WIGS

Replica, Lady's wig, c. 1774
Replica, Grizzled man's wig, c. 1774
Colonial Williamsburg Foundation

Replica of c. 1750 gentleman's
powdered wig
Replica of c. 1780 gentleman's
powdered wig
New York State Museum, Albany,
New York

Wig of Harpo Marx, c. 1930
Wig of Bozo the Clown, c. 1960
Wig of Celia Cruz, c. 1980
National Museum of American
History, Behring Center, Smithsonian
Institution

HAIR STYLING TOOLS AND PRODUCTS

Collection of shaving tools including razors, strops, brushes, and comfort kit, early 20th century
Dimensions variable
New York State Military Museum and Veterans Research Center, Saratoga Springs, New York

Collection of hair styling tools including curling irons, hair dryers, crimpers, and receivers; hair styling products including powders, dyes, pomades, restorers, and shampoos; and shaving tools including razors, strops, and mugs, 19th and 20th centuries
Permanent Wave machine, early 20th century
Beauty salon chair with attached dryer hood, mid-20th century
Barber's chair with child's extra seat, c. 1930
Dimensions variable
New York State Museum, Albany, New York

Gillette "Khaki Set" U.S. Army Issue, 1917–18
Razor, blades, mirror, box
2 x 4 1/4 x 1 3/4 inches

Imperial Rolls Razor No. 2
Blade, hone, strop, strop dressing
2 x 6 3/4 inches
Collection of Virginia Gooch Puzak, Skidmore Class of 1944

Barber's vest of Nathaniel Mathis (Nat the Bush Doctor), c. 1970
curling iron set, razor
Dimensions variable
National Museum of American History, Behring Center, Smithsonian Institution

Collection of hair styling tools
Dimensions variable
Collection of Bonny Thornton, Wilton, New York

Hot oil hair staightening comb, 1950s
9 1/4 x 1 1/4 x 1 inches
Collection of David Rubin, New York

ADVERTISEMENTS

Breck Girl (Donna Alexander), 1974
16 3/8 x 13 3/8 inches

Hall's Hair Renewer and Buckingham's Dye
14 x 11 1/2 inches

Hall's Hair Renewer
13 7/8 x 11 inches

Dr. Dickes' Shampoo
15 x 12 1/4 inches

Brass Hair Straightening Combs and Pressers
11 5/8 x 11 1/8 inches

Seven Sutherland Sisters' Hair Grower
9 x 11 1/2 inches

Colgate's Shaving Lather
13 3/8 x 10 1/2 inches

Gillette Safety Razor
14 1/8 x 9 3/8 inches

Madam Jones Seven X Hot Comb Oil
3 3/4 x 7 1/8 inches

Sweet Georgia Brown Hair Glower
1 5/8 x 6 1/8 inches

Burma Shave
Paint on wooden boards
40 x 18 1/4 inches each
National Museum of American History, Behring Center, Smithsonian Institution

PRINTS

ANONYMOUS

Mlle. des Faveurs à la Promenade à Londres, 18th century
Hand-colored etching
13 1/2 x 10 15/16 inches
Print Collection, Miriam and Ira D. Wallach Division of Art, Prints and Photographs, The New York Public Library, Astor, Lenox and Tilden Foundations

WILLIAM HOGARTH

A Midnight Modern Conversation, 1732–33
Etching and engraving
13 1/2 x 18 5/8 inches
Print Collection, Miriam and Ira D. Wallach Division of Art, Prints and Photographs, The New York Public Library, Astor, Lenox and Tilden Foundations

The Bench, 1758
Etching and engraving
13 1/2 x 9 1/4 inches
The Tang Teaching Museum, Skidmore College, Gift of Edwin de Turck Bechtel, 1957.50

The Five Orders of Periwigs, 1761
Etching and engraving
12 1/4 x 9 inches
The Tang Teaching Museum,
Skidmore College, Gift of Edwin de
Turck Bechtel, ND.109

Published by **WILLIAM HUMPHREY**
Beauty's Lot, n.d.
Engraving
12 3/4 x 7 7/8 inches
Library of Congress, Washington,
D.C., Prints and Photographs Division

PHILIP DAWE
The Enraged Macaroni, 1773
Mezzotint
12 5/8 x 9 3/4 inches
Library of Congress, Washington,
D.C., Prints and Photographs Division

*The Macaroni. A Real Character at
the Late Masquerade*, 1773
Mezzotint
13 7/8 x 10 inches
Print Collection, Miriam and
Ira D. Wallach Division of Art, Prints
and Photographs, The New York
Public Library, Astor, Lenox and
Tilden Foundations

Published by **R. SAYER & J.
BENNETT**
What Is This My Son Tom, 1774
Mezzotint
13 7/8 x 9 7/8 inches
Library of Congress, Washington,
D.C., Prints and Photographs Division

Published by **MATTHEW AND
MARY DARLY**
*Oh Heigh Oh – Or a View of the
Back Settlements*, 1776
Engraving
13 7/8 x 9 7/8 inches
Library of Congress, Washington,
D.C., Prints and Photographs Division

*The Vis a Vis Bisected, or the Ladies'
Coop*, 1776
Etching and engraving
9 3/4 x 13 3/4 inches
Print Collection, Miriam and
Ira D. Wallach Division of Art, Prints
and Photographs, The New York
Public Library, Astor, Lenox and
Tilden Foundations

Published by **W. HUMPHREY**
*The Modern Paradise or Adam and
Eve Regenerated*, 1780
Etching
9 3/4 x 3 3/4 inches
Library of Congress, Washington,
D.C., Prints and Photographs Division

ISAAC CRUIKSHANK
Ladies Wigs!, 1798
Hand-colored etching
14 3/8 x 19 1/2 inches
Print Collection, Miriam and
Ira D. Wallach Division of Art, Prints
and Photographs, The New York
Public Library, Astor, Lenox and
Tilden Foundations

EDWARD WILLIAM STODART
Lolita, 19th century
Stiple engraving
17 3/4 x 13 inches
The Tang Teaching Museum,
Skidmore College, ND.184

Sweet Little Mary Pickford, 1914
13 3/4 x 10 5/8 inches

Coquette, 1928
12 3/16 x 9 1/8 inches
National Museum of American
History, Behring Center, Smithsonian
Institution

FEDERICO CASTELLÓN
From the *Masque of the Red Death*
series, 20th century
Lithograph
15 x 11 inches
The Tang Teaching Museum,
Skidmore College, 1969.14.1

PHOTOGRAPHS

CHARLES EISENMANN
Illumara the Egyptian, Age 19, c. 1860
Albumen print carte-de-visite
International Center of Photography,
New York

ANONYMOUS
Unidentified Portraits, c. 1920
Gelatin-silver prints
International Center of Photography,
New York

ROBERT CAPA
Nazi Conspirators, 1944–45
Gelatin-silver print
International Center of Photography,
New York

BRUCE DAVIDSON
Brooklyn Gang, 1959
Gelatin-silver print
8 1/4 x 12 1/2 inches
International Center of Photography,
New York

PHILIPPE HALSMAN
Portrait of Marilyn, 1952
(from "Halsman/Marilyn," 1981)
Gelatin-silver print
11 x 8 1/2 inches
Williams College Museum of Art,
Gift of Marjorie Neikrug-Raskin

GARY METZ
Hair Piece, 1977
Twenty gelatin-silver prints
14 x 11 inches each
Courtesy of the artist

CARRIE MAE WEEMS
Snow White-Mirror Mirror, 1987
Gelatin-silver print
20 x 16 inches
On extended loan to the Tang Teaching
Museum from a private collection

JEANNE DUNNING
Head 8, 1990
Laminated cibachrome mounted
on plexiglass
30 x 19 inches
On extended loan to the Tang Teaching
Museum from a private collection

STEPHAN CARAS
Victor Trevmo in Swan Lake, Act II,
1997
Color photograph
19 1/4 x 15 inches
National Museum of Dance and Hall
of Fame, Saratoga Springs, New York

VIK MUNIZ
Medusa Marinara, 1999
Photograph on plate
12 1/2 inches diameter
On extended loan to the Tang Teaching
Museum from a private collection

BOOKS

LOUIS DU GUERNIER AND
CLAUDE DU BOSC
Illustration for canto III, from
Alexander Pope, *Rape of the Lock*,
1714
7 1/2 x 4 3/4 inches
Special Collection of the Schaffer
Library at Union College

HEINRICH HOFFMAN
*Der Struwwelpeter, oder lustige
Geschichten und drollige Bilder*, 1845
Collection of Mary Constance Lynn,
Saratoga Springs, New York

*Slovenly Peter or Cheerful Stories and
Funny Pictures*, 20th century
Collection of John Anzalone,
Saratoga Springs, New York

Godey's Fashions for February 1864
from *Godey's Magazine*, February
1864
Special Collection of the Lucy
Scribner Library at Skidmore College

DANTE GABRIEL ROSSETTI
*Buy From Us With a Golden Curl and
Golden Head by Golden Head*
from Christina Rossetti, *Goblin
Market and Other Poems*, 1862
6 1/2 x 4 1/4 inches
Special Collection of the Schaffer
Library at Union College

Godey's Fashions for July 1864
from *Godey's Magazine*, July 1864
Special Collection of the Lucy
Scribner Library at Skidmore College

GUSTAVE DORÉ
Samson and Delilah and *Penitent
Mary Magdalene*,
from *La Sainte Bible*, 1874
Special Collection of the Lucy
Scribner Library at Skidmore College

AUBREY BEARDSLEY
Illustration for "J'ai Baisé ta Bouche,
Iokanaan," from Oscar Wilde,
Salome: A Tragedy in One Act, 1894
Collection of John Anzalone,
Saratoga Springs, New York

The Comedy of the Rhinegold
from *The Savoy*, December 1896
Special Collection of the Lucy
Scribner Library at Skidmore College

The Rape of the Lock
from *The Savoy*, April 1896
Special Collection of the Lucy Scribner
Library at Skidmore College

RALPH BARTON
Illustration for *But a Diamond
Bracelet Lasts Forever*,
from Anita Loos, *Gentlemen Prefer
Blondes: The Illuminating Diary of a
Professional Lady*, 1925
7 1/4 x 5 inches
Collection of the Schaffer Library at
Union College

Compiled by **LEIGH HUNT**
Hair of Famous Writers (Elizabeth
Barrett Browning, Robert Browning,
John Keats, Richard Henry Lee,
John Milton, Mary Shelley, Percy
Bysshe Shelley, George Washington)
Human hair, prints
Each page 14 1/2 x 10 3/4 inches
Harry Ransom Center, University of
Texas at Austin

ACKNOWLEDGMENTS

Hair: Untangling a Social History began as an idea from Professor Penny Jolly for a project at the museum that would look at the many facets of hair imagery and its ramifications throughout western culture. To condense this imposingly large topic, Prof. Jolly organized a senior week symposium at the Tang Museum in the spring of 2002. The symposium was a full day of presentations from a variety of Skidmore faculty that included papers on the biochemistry, anthropology, literary history, art history, and sociology of human hair. These engaging talks, often punctuated with hilariously be-wigged presenters, helped form the content of this catalogue and exhibition.

The exhibition includes objects from a wide variety of sources, from Final Touch Hair Salon to the Smithsonian Institution, and we are very grateful to the many individuals and institutions that helped locate materials, offered advice, and generously loaned us their objects. Thanks to: Adam Weinberg, Susan Faxon, Denise Johnson, James M. Sousa, Addison Gallery of American Art, Phillips Academy, Andover, Massachusetts; Christine Miles, Tammis Groft, Mary Alice Mackey, Diane Shewchuck, Sarah Bennet, Albany Institute of History & Art, Albany, New York; Kathy Gaye Shiroki, Albright-Knox Art Gallery, Buffalo, New York; John Anzalone, Skidmore College; Alfred L. Chatelain, L'Epoque Romantique, French and American Antiques, Queensbury, New York; Ruth Copans, Nancy Rudick, Lucy Scribner Library, Skidmore College; Tim Wiles, W.C. Burdick, National Baseball Hall of Fame and Museum, Cooperstown, New York; Michael Conforti, Brian Allen, Monique LeBlanc, Katherine Price, The Sterling and Francine Clark Art Institute, Williamstown, Massachusetts; Elizabeth Myers, Thomas E. Redd, Colonial Williamsburg Foundation, Williamsburg, Virginia; Susan Crossley and Timothy Collins, San Francisco, California; Volker Diehl, Annkatrin Steffen, Galerie Volker Diehl, Berlin, Germany; Beverly and Warren Daniel, Wayland, Massachusetts; Ms. Lori Gladstone, Baltimore, Maryland; Robin Graham, Cameron M. Shay, Priscilla Vail Caldwell, Marisa Mele, James Graham & Sons Gallery, New York; Mrs. Nancy Hirsche, Sarasota, Florida; Erin Doan, Historical Society of Saratoga Springs, New York; Randall Suffolk, Erin Coe, Robin Blakney-Carlson, The Hyde Collection, Glens Falls, New York; Willis E. Hartshorn, Barbara Woytowicz, Cynthia Young, International Center of Photography, New York, New York; Howard Fox, Nancy Thomas, Michele Ahern, Cheryle T. Robertson, Giselle Arteaga-Johnson, Los Angeles County Museum of Art, Los Angeles, California; Sara W. Duke, Margaret Brown, Library of Congress, Washington, D.C.; Mary Constance Lynn, Skidmore College; Gavin McKeirnan, Gary Metz, Providence, Rhode Island; Malcolm Rogers, Elliot Bostwick Davis, Kim Pashko, Lisabeth Dion, Annie Pickert, Courtney Peterson, Museum of Fine Arts, Boston, Massachusetts; David Shayt, Shelly Foote, Lisa Graddy, Fath Ruffins, Dwight Bowers, Roger White, Pat Mansfield, Lynne Gilliland, Carol Slatick, Margaret Grandine, Kay Peterson, Dave Burgevin, Smithsonian Institution, National Museum of American History, Washington, D.C.; Garret Smith, National Museum of Dance, Saratoga Springs, New York; Roberta Waddell, Roseann Panebianco, Tom LeSante, The New York Public Library, New York; Michael Aikey, Christopher Morton, New York State Military Museum and Veterans Research Center, Saratoga Springs, New York; Anne Tyrrell, Ronald Burch, Craig Williams, Geoffrey Stein, New York State Museum, Albany, New York; Debra Priestly, New York, New York; Virginia Gooch Puzak, Skidmore College Class of 1944; Gregory Perry, Cathleen Anderson, Linda Strandberg, Jane Voorhees Zimmerli Art Museum, Rutgers, State University of New Jersey, New Brunswick, New Jersey; Bonny Thornton, Final Touch Beauty Salon, Wilton, New York; Paul Tucker; Julianna Spallholz, Schaffer Library, Union College, Schenectady, New York; Tara Wenger, David Coleman, Deborah R. Armstrong-Morgan, Harry Ransom Humanities Research Center, The University of Texas at Austin; David Rubin; Jack Shainman; Gordon Thompson, Skidmore College; Linda Shearer, Vivian Patterson, Stephanie Jandl, Diane Hart, Williams College Museum of Art, Williamstown, Massachusetts; Amy Meyers, Timothy Goodhue, Melissa G. Fournier, Yale Center for British Art, New Haven, Connecticut; and an anonymous private collector. Special thanks to Skidmore students Emily Shultz, Stephanie Greene, and Haley Cohen, who assisted with research.

Important support from the Gillette Corporation and the Nathalie Potter Voorhees '45 memorial fund have made this project possible. Also thanks to the Office of the Dean of the Faculty at Skidmore College, and to the Faculty Development Committee who awarded this project a Tang Exhibition Award. Thanks to Barry Pritzker, Stephanie Van Allen, Mary Jo Driscoll, Tracy Barlok, Barbara Melville, and Elizabeth Laub, also at Skidmore.

This catalogue includes new essays by several faculty members whose engaging contributions exemplify the potential of a teaching museum as a site for interdisciplinary collaboration. Thanks to Gerald Erchak, Professor of Anthropology at Skidmore College; Amelia Rauser, Associate Professor of Art History at Franklin and Marshall College; Jeffrey Segrave, Professor of Exercise Science and Director of Athletics at Skidmore; and Susan Walzer, Associate Professor of Sociology at Skidmore. The design of this volume is the creative work of graphic designers Barbara Glauber and Beverly Joel of Heavy Meta, New York. Thanks to Arthur Evans for his new photography and Kathryn Gallien for her keen editing.

As always the entire Tang Museum staff has contributed greatly to the success of this project. Special thanks are due to former Director Charles Stainback for his early support and important creative work on this project; Elizabeth Karp, Registrar, who managed the shipping of the many loans; Chris Kobuskie, Chief Preparator, for his work framing and building the exhibition; Susi Kerr, Assistant Director for Education and Public Programs, who managed the many lectures, films and events held in conjunction with this project and Ginny Kollack who recorded "Hair Clips" from many members of the Skidmore community. Also thanks to staff members: Tyler Auwarter, Helaina Blume, Jill Cohan, Ginger Ertz, Lori Geraghty, Gayle King, Barbara Schrade, and our installation crew: Sam Coe, Shaw Fici, Torrance Fish, Jefferson Nelson, Patrick O' Rourke, Chris Oliver, Alex Roediger, and Joe Yetto.

Curatorial Assistant Gretchen Wagner deserves great thanks for her tireless work on all aspects of this complex and detailed project. She visited with lenders, managed loans, organized reproductions, and attended to everything in between. The project would not have been possible without her savvy and determination.

Lastly, thanks to guest curator, Penny Jolly. Professor Jolly is the William R. Kenan Chair of Liberal Arts and Professor of Art History at Skidmore College. She has served as curator, researcher, writer, and editor, and has paved the way for future ambitious projects at the Tang. Her concept to look at images of hair and the cultural implications that inform those images fits perfectly with our mission as a museum based on ideas, and this exhibition and catalogue show how those ideas can open the door to many disciplines. We are most grateful for her intellectual engagement and her energy that has made this project a great success.

IAN BERRY
Associate Director for Curatorial Affairs/Curator

This catalogue accompanies the exhibition

HAIR: UNTANGLING A SOCIAL HISTORY

January 31–June 6, 2004

The Tang Teaching Museum and Art Gallery
Skidmore College
815 North Broadway
Saratoga Springs, New York 12866
T 518 580 8080
F 518 580 5069
www.skidmore.edu/tang

©2004 The Frances Young Tang Teaching Museum and
Art Gallery

ISBN 0-9725188-3-5

Catalogue Editor: Ian Berry
Text Editor: Kathryn Gallien

Designed by Barbara Glauber and Beverly Joel
Heavy Meta

Printed in the United States by
John C. Otto Company, Inc.

Photograph Credits
Plates 1, 8, 25: Addison Gallery of American Art,
Phillips Academy, Andover, Massachusetts. All rights
reserved, photographs by Gerg Heins.
Plates 2, 5, 11, 12, 13, 14, 15, 26, 28, 29, 31, 33, 40, 41, 44,
47, 48: photographs by Arthur Evans.
Plate 3: Yale Center for British Art, New Haven,
Connecticut, photo by Richard Caspole
Plate 4: photo by Michael Fredericks.
Plates 6, 24: Addison Gallery of American Art,
Phillips Academy, Andover, Massachusetts.
All rights reserved, photographs by the Williamstown
Art Conservation Center.
Plates 7, 38, 39: Albany Institute of History & Art, Albany,
New York.
Plate 9: Photograph ©2003, Museum of Fine Arts, Boston
Plates 10, 27, 49, 53: National Museum of American
History, Behring Center, Smithsonian Institution,
Washington D.C., images by Kay Peterson.
Plates 16, 19, 20, 21: New York Public Library, New York,
New York.
Plates 17, 18, 22: The Library of Congress, Washington,
D.C.
Plate 23: photo by Steven Sloman.
Plates 30, 51: National Museum of American History,
Behring Center, Smithsonian Institution, Washington
D.C., images by Dave Burgevin.
Plate 32: Courtesy of Adam Baumgold Gallery, New York
Plate 34: Sterling and Francine Clark Art Institute,
Williamstown, Massachusetts.
Plates 35–37: The Harry Ransom Humanities Research
Center, University of Texas at Austin, Austin, Texas.
Plate 42: Jane Voorhees Zimmerli Art Museum,
Rutgers State University of New Jersey, New Brunswick,
New Jersey.
Plate 43: Galerie Volker Diehl, Berlin, photo by Jurgen
Baumann.
Plate 45: Williams College Museum of Art, Williamstown,
Massachusetts.
Plate 46: Courtesy of Lori Gladstone.
Plate 50: Los Angeles County Museum of Art, Los
Angeles, California 2003 Museum Associates/LACMA.
Plate 52: Courtesy of Debra Priestly, photo by Manu
Sassoonian.